TEENAGE ADDICTS
CAN RECOVER

Treating The Addict, Not The Age

Shelly Marshall

GYLANTIC PUBLISHING COMPANY
LITTLETON, COLORADO

Although the author has extensively researched all information to ensure the accuracy and completeness of the information contained in this book, the author and publisher assume no responsibility for errors inaccuracies, omissions or any other inconsistency herein. Data contained herein are the most complete and accurate available as this book goes to print. Please bear in mind that meanings can vary due to personal interpretation.

To order additional copies:

GYLANTIC PUBLISHING COMPANY
P.O Box 2792
Littleton, Colorado 80161-2792   (303)797-6093

Library of Congress Cataloging-in-Publication Data

Marshall, Shelly.
   Teenage addicts can recover : treating the addict, not the age / Shelly Marshall.
      p.   cm.
   Includes index.
   ISBN 1-880197-02-2 : $12.95
   1. Teenagers—United States—Alcohol use. 2. Teenagers—United States—Drug use. 3. Alcoholics—Rehabilitation—United States. 4. Narcotic addicts—Rehabilitation—United States. 5. Teenagers-
-Counseling of—United States. I. Title.
HV5135.M3655 1992
362.29'2'0835—dc20   92-19282
                                                        CIP

Table of Contents

Foreword

It seems like every other news story is related to the terrible effects of drugs—crack addiction, drunk driving, and drug wars, to name a few. Questions arise in the curious minds of our four kids as they watch this panoply of horror flash across the nightly news. "What are drugs Daddy? What do they do to people? Why do some kids take them?" they ask. My answer always seems to come out more maudlin than one would expect from a professional psychologist, "Drugs are bad. They destroy lives." I am desperately trying to inoculate my kids from future drug addiction. My biggest fear is that they may succumb to the evil allure of mind altering chemicals, a fear that is not unfounded given my family history—a veritable graveyard littered with the wreckage of alcoholism and drug abuse. Just about everyone today has a personal reason for being concerned about drug addiction.

I'm sorry to say that as far as I know, no one has come up with an answer to the problem of drug abuse. But fortunately, the outlook is not all bleak. There are a few rays of hope — compassionate and dedicated professionals are devoting their lives to working in the field of chemical dependency and recovery. I am proud to say that my sister, Shelly Marshall, is one of those dedicated professionals. She has devoted her life to understanding how chemically dependent teenagers can best recover. Her accomplishments in the field are numerous. She graduated from

Metropolitan State College in Denver with the first BS degree awarded in Human Services with a speciality: Drugs and Alcohol. She then went on to earn a ThB degree in counseling from Burton College and Seminary in Denver. This theoretical knowledge was put to work by spending eight years as a staff therapist for teenage alcoholics in recovery programs at such places as the General Hospital and St. Lukes Hospital in Denver. Shelly went on to co-found two recovery programs: The Hand of Hope, a halfway home for recovering young people, and the Cortez Community Mission detox center. Her books *Day By Day, Young, Sober, & Free* and *Teenage Addicts Can Recover* with combined sales approaching the 2 1/2 million have enabled her to have a significant impact in the area of adolescent addiction recovery. Now her new book *Teenage Addicts Can Recover* explores important information for those working with addicted teens. In addition she has published the results of several scientific studies in journals like *The International Journal Of The Addictions* and *The American Journal Of Alcohol And Drug Abuse*.

Does all this qualify her as an expert in the field of addiction recovery? No. Not without the personal knowledge that can only be derived from suffering through three generations of drug abuse. As I know all too well, she is an adult child of an alcoholic. Our parents are both alcoholic. She recovered from the disease at age twenty-one and now is the mother of an eighteen year-old daughter, who also is trying to recover from alcohol and drug abuse.

Teenagers, in their youthful brashness, are notoriously difficult for recovery personnel to reach. According to research studies their recidivism rate is significantly higher than that of adults. In an attempt to mollify themselves, some recovery professionals subscribe to the "we planted a seed" theory. They tell themselves, "The addicts know where to come back for help when they are ready to stop using." This belief is fraught with hazards. Too many teens will die before they make it back to help. The family of these teens will pay too heavy a price for delayed recovery. Can we expect more from teenage recovery programs? Shelly Marshall believes the answer is yes. She proposes a model of recovery which has the goal of raising the teenage recovery success rate to that of the better programs for adults. In this book she offers these insights to all who might care to listen.

Michael J. Marshall, Ph.D., Assistant Professor of Psychology
North Carolina A & T State University

Section I

Assessment Phase

Introduction

This section examines pre-treatment areas of concern for parents, schools and professionals involved in adolescent alcoholism and other drug addictions. Those trying desperately to save the lives of teenagers will get a new look at some of the basic assumptions in the field.

Since the study of teenage alcoholism/addiction is in its infancy, there is little research to draw on in reaching the drug-affected adolescent. In order to avoid using outdated models such as crisis lines and comic book literature, professionals must turn to the extensive body of research on adult addiction in seeking answers.

The first four chapters examine those pre-treatment issues with a fresh approach. Chapter 1 cautions parents who suspect drug abuse to seek assessment help from professionals trained specifically in the field of addiction. Parents should not rely solely upon the advice of such non-expert authorities as teachers, ministers or police. Certain thinking traps may prevent parents from recognizing the severity or even existence of their child's drug use. Lastly, parents are asked to be aware of and support those laws and programs that allow them some control over the direction of their teenagers' lives.

Chapter 2 presents some key concepts that will help parents make informed decisions about how and where to get the best recovery help for their addicted adolescent. Chapter 3 examines basic questions about teenage drug addiction, such as, "Is alcoholism really a psychological problem, a family problem or a disease?" Finally, Chapter 4 identifies and discusses the hidden prejudices professionals and others may harbor about teenage addicts.

The pre-treatment concepts in this section are derived from the work and findings of innovative professionals in the field, the adult alcoholism literature, and personal research. Using these concepts to assess and refer teenage addicts will lay the foundation for successful treatment.

Chapter 1

Identifying the Troubled Teen

In the Sixties, the problem of teenage addiction exploded across this nation. Since then volumes have been written about teenagers and drug abuse. Yet the impact of teenage drug abuse is greater today than ever. Children are using at younger ages, starting in grammar school. Teenagers are experimenting with dangerous chemicals like crack and designer drugs and are craftier at deceiving school officials and parents.

Most parents are not easily deceived about their children's use of drugs, but the greater the degree of drug abuse, the greater their denial. Even the most educated parents succumb to this form of self-protection. "I've brought my child up right. I know he'll rationally consider his choices." Or "Not my kid—she's too smart, too young, loves God too much, is close to me, etc...." Or "I am teaching my kid how to drink responsibly so he won't have problems."

No parent wants a child abusing drugs. No school system wants its students dying from addiction. No court system invites the crimes generated from the disease and abuse of mind altering-chemicals. But often, when individuals such as parents, teachers, or parole officers push to bring awareness to our neighborhoods, school districts, and communities, they meet with resistance.

This resistance to awareness is born of fear. It is human nature to subconsciously think, *If I ignore it, it won't be there.* Now, with all the media attention and efforts of public awareness campaigns from the "Just Say No" ads to the National Council on Alcoholism's programs, alcoholism/addiction is difficult to ignore. So the human response to this is, "It might be in that neighborhood, but doesn't affect us here."

This human resistance is exemplified by a mother in Whitewater, Wisconsin. Jean Sable went to extraordinary measures to help her drug-abusing son. This mother became an expert on her son's problem. Jean wrote papers on alcoholism and addiction and had them published. She spoke to groups, involved herself in community endeavors to promote education, set up workshops, served on drug and alcohol awareness boards, worked on a hot line, and counseled women with chemical problems for the Employee Assistance Program at the University of Wisconsin, Whitewater.

Jean's involvement is impressive. Yet for all this mother's dedication to helping her son she has this to say about her community:

> No matter how hard I and many others who shared my concerns worked, we did not seem to be able to create awareness about this problem or to gain support for needed preventive programs in our communities.
>
> My son's chemical dependency continued through high school and he refused all the help my husband and I tried to give him. Within a five-year period, seven of my son's friends had died from what was then termed "experimenting with chemicals." When the seventh boy died, I vowed I would find a way to show the people who said, "There is nothing you can do," that they were wrong.
>
> Seven kids died in a five-year period in a very small community. Yet the community still looked the other way and said that it wasn't a real problem in their town. When it becomes obvious that drugs are a real problem in a community, the rationalization transforms to, "It's not a real problem in our family."

This was the response Jean encountered when she tried to help other parents identify and do something about the drug problem in Whitewater. After the seventh adolescent died, a situation occurred which prompted Jean to try again to reach other parents. A particularly wild unauthorized party was thrown by her son while Jean and her husband were gone for the day. When they returned, the police informed the couple about the party and that various drugs were found in their house. Jean took action:

> I contacted the parents of every young person I thought might have been in our home. I did not ask them to come, I begged them.

> Some parents came to my home and I am sorry to say not much was accomplished. We were confronted with an enormous amount of denial, the desire to find someone, or something to blame and a search for quick, easy answers. One couple was furious we even had the meeting. They were modern, well-educated parents. They happened to know for a fact that all young people were going to experiment with chemicals. Big deal. A little pot, a little speed, a little booze isn't going to hurt anybody. It's a fad, just forget it, don't overreact. Another couple grinned and poked each other and finally the mother said, "Jean, our son is such a neat kid. Even though he knew he'd be punished, he admitted he skipped school and went to the party. But he only goes to those parties to observe. He likes to watch other children drink and get high and stuff. He wouldn't do it." The last woman said, "Well, all we really have to do is find the fink pusher in Whitewater, nail that sucker to a cross and our problems are over, because we won't have any chemicals."

> After the parents left my home that night, we went in different directions and we did all the wrong things for the right reasons. And, we learned that our children were right about one thing—we didn't know what we were talking about. We didn't know that by the time their behavior had deteriorated to the point that we could see something was wrong—our kids were already lying, cheating, stealing and dealing.

How do we know our children are already lying, stealing and dealing? It's simple. It's common sense. Drug and alcohol use is illegal. So, even to experiment, teenagers have to start lying. Consider the expense: eventually they have to cheat, steal and deal to get the drugs. Whether they steal it from your liquor cabinet, take money from your purse, rob others, or sell sexual favors—adolescents do not have the resources to support any continuing drug use without resorting to immoral and illegal activities.

So how do we identify the drug-using behavior before it reaches the final stages? How do we identify the problem before the young girl is walking the streets, before our son is selling crack from his locker, before several kids die in a gang shooting, before a friend's child dies in a drunk-driving accident, before a child takes a deadly overdose? The first step, of course, is education. Our society has made major strides in this area. We have many public awareness campaigns. Nancy Reagan (despite all the flaws in her approach) has helped us a great deal. Schools are adopting education programs for our children. Even private treatment centers, however self-serving in nature, have used commercial time to open the eyes of the public to the proximity and vastness of the problem.

But education does not eliminate the problem. It only makes it visible. Once the problem is visible the community and parents must acknowledge the problem and accept the challenge to make change.

Ironically, it is at this point that parents face a lot of frustrations or *Dead Ends*. If you have read this far in the book, you are educating yourself. Now you will begin to face the DEAD ENDS so many confront when beginning to recognize the problems in our communities, schools, and kids.

DEAD END NUMBER 1:

School systems are often confused about their role in student alcoholism/addiction and will ignore issues rather than risk doing the wrong thing.

The most likely people to notice a teenager's problem with drugs and alcohol are parents and teachers. Teachers and other school staff need to be alert to the symptoms of drug use—not to diagnose—but to observe and record behavior and request evaluations. Teachers must be responsible for noticing changes and problems, but not for diagnosing disease, counseling troubled teens or bringing about changes in their lives.

Rick Swords, public relations spokesman for New Beginnings in Lakewood, Colorado, says:

> I can't ask teachers to diagnose, educate, counsel, and/or correct all problems. They haven't got the time if they want to teach. So I (we) ask them to simply record impaired behavior. Observe and record. Then if a certain number of problem indicators crop up, we ask them to request an evaluation. The evaluation is done by the school psychologist or counselor, using the observations of the teacher and school records, and this evaluation is then discussed with the student and his parents. If

drugs are implicated they call me or any treatment center liaison and we do a more comprehensive evaluation with school, parents, and student.

We need to eliminate the teacher's and school's liability. As long as they are not labeling kids as addicts or abusers or mentally ill, they will not have to face irate parents, demanding parent-teacher groups, or even lawsuits. They will be freer to spot and report trouble if they won't be called on the carpet for it.

A generic type Impaired Behavior Worksheet (Figure 1 is an example of such a form) could lead to any number of conclusions, and not all drug-related. The pattern of facts and impressions documented on this worksheet might expose physical or sexual abuse in the family, signs of mental illness or learning disabilities. Perhaps it documents rebellion well within the normal range for this stage of development. But it may also reveal the beginning stages of a teenager's alcoholism/addiction.

The evaluation process begins with the instructors. When they become concerned over a student's appearance, behavior, attitude, or choice of friends, they record their observations and send the form to the school office. The office adds data from their student files and passes the form to the school psychologist or counselor. After interviewing the student, the counselor arranges a family conference including the student, and makes final evaluations.

The group—counselor, parents, and student—decide what is to be done. Does the teen need special education support, medical or psychological help, or chemical dependency treatment? After this evaluation, the student is referred to a specialist for diagnosis and treatment. The teacher or counselor is not asked for a diagnosis only to observe behavior and record. A teacher or counselor should never be asked for a professional diagnosis.

This program of evaluation is easy to implement in any school system. A workshop to familiarize faculty with the procedure could be completed in about an hour. It requires no special training or funding and most private treatment centers have school liaisons who would be able to help.

Figure 1.

IMPAIRED BEHAVIOR WORKSHEET

Date_____

I,_____, am requesting an evaluation of _____
_____ because I am concerned for him/her as a result of
observing the following behaviors:

IS THE STUDENT?

a) Missing assignments, especially those to be done over the weekend or
on holidays

Remark_____

b) Falling asleep in class or having frequent lapses in concentration

Remark_____

c) Frequent tardiness or early departure from class

Remark_____

d) Evidence of chemical abuse: alcohol on the breath, slurred speech,
poor balance, odor of marijuana, etc.

Remark_____

e) Depression, undue agitation, particularly belligerent and/or violent
attitudes and actions

Remark_____

f) Other

Remark_____

FOR OFFICE USE:

a) Is this student associating with the identified drinking and drug crowd
or known dealers?

Remark_____

b) Have drug paraphernalia been noted on student or in his locker?

Remark_____

c) Is student often absent, tardy, truant, absent on Mondays, or have many unexcused absences?

Remark_____

d) Is student often sick, making frequent trips to the school nurse for vague symptoms?

Remark_____

e) Has disciplinary action been necessary?

Remark_____

FOR THE COUNSELOR OR SCHOOL PSYCHOLOGIST:

a) Does student drink and/or use drugs/alcohol?

Remark_____

b) Is there a family history of alcohol and drug abuse in parent, extended family, siblings?

Remark_____

c) Does student have symptoms of depression or potential for suicide: isolation, past suicide attempts, threats of suicide, self-destructive behavior, cutting or scratching self, constant fighting?

Remark_____

d) Has student been involved with police through arrests, detention, or jail time?

Remark_____

e) Are the parents concerned about the child? What do they suspect?

Remark_____

f) Is the student concerned about himself? What does he or she suspect is causing the problem?

Remark_____

There is more than one way of evaluating student behavior for potential drug abuse. Each school system is unique and involves different personalities, administrative structures, and state laws. Contacting the school counselor or drug specialist is a good place to begin. Emphasize that screening requires no special training, no funding, and eliminates all liability of the school and teachers. More importantly screening is a positive action they can take with troubled students.

DEAD END NUMBER 2:

When responsible parents try to get help, they often find their hands are tied.

By whom? By the legal system, by the school system, by judgmental neighbors. It is almost impossible to force a child to do anything. Most types of discipline are now seen as child abuse. In many states, if a parent leaves any type of red mark, however small, the schools are required to report the incident to the authorities. Most state laws stipulate that parents cannot physically restrain a child or use physical force to require children to do anything, including going to a psychologist, doctor, or obtaining treatment for addiction.

There are self-proclaimed experts claiming that even using a loud voice is a form of abuse. Social service systems, in some instances, have gotten so out of hand as to enable the addict. Some parents are actually frightened that their children will have them put in jail. Children learn the system very fast: basically they can do what they want and parents are powerless to stop them.

The following example points out the difficult parents can experience in working with the social system. One woman has been fighting a terrific battle trying to deal with a state department that, in protecting her child, has turned her family into a war zone.

My daughter decided she was angry at me and my husband, her stepdad. My daughter heard from another girl at school that if she said my husband was molesting her, welfare would take her out of the home. She "turned him in" and we lost custody based on my child's confused testimony. Nothing was verified either legally or medically.

My girl had been pretty sweet up to this point. Finally Sherry wanted to come home and admitted to her sister that she lied to hurt us.

After a medical examination, it was shown she was a virgin and what she'd accused my husband of didn't seem to be true.

In the meantime, welfare taught Sherry her "rights" and insisted she stay in group therapy. Sherry never wanted to go and begged out of the sessions all the time. Later I discovered she was still telling welfare that my husband did molest her and I wouldn't believe her. My daughter also told her therapy group that I wouldn't drive her and that's why she wouldn't come. When welfare confronted her, she said, "I told Mom I didn't want to go to make it easy on her." Sherry tells everyone a different story. She used to mind me. Now she threatens to "turn me in" any time I ask her to behave. I cry all the time; I don't know what or whom to believe anymore. Welfare became my enemy in the guise of protecting my daughter from her stepfather and me. Why aren't we working together to help my girl? Why aren't we together, trying to discover the truth? Not as enemies...

It is not unusual for parents to recognize problems in their children and find that they cannot require them to get help, go to school after age sixteen, restrain them from getting drugs, or even kick them out of the house if their child does not want to go. Often all a child has to do is claim "abuse" of any kind and some welfare departments decide the parents are adversarial and engage in "battle" before the facts are known.

To make matters worse, laws are decriminalizing drunkenness without proposing standards for treatment. Recently, the state of Washington passed a law decriminalizing drunkenness in minors. It is illegal for a child to buy or drink alcohol but not to have it in the bloodstream, so if a police officer sees a child staggering around drunkenly, he can do nothing. The child has to be in possession of the alcohol. No one can figure out what the legislators had in mind—not the police and not the parents. But the kids think it is a big joke on the authorities. It is legal for them to be drunk.

In Wisconsin, a new law has been enacted for minors. Referred to as "Not a Drop" law, it demands that minors caught driving with any blood alcohol content automatically lose their license for a period of time. Wisconsin legislators feel that if it is illegal for a minor to drink, then it is illegal for a minor to drive with even a drop of alcohol in the blood. This law supports the rule that forbids teens to use alcohol.

There are two solutions to the powerlessness of this *Dead End*. One is political. Support laws and school policies that support parents. Legal and

social attitudes which automatically cast parents as the "bad guys" need
to be balanced. In the meantime work within the available system and
make changes where possible.

The second is to take a "tough love" type of approach. This method is
taught in many communities and is described in literature available from
local branches of the National Council on Alcoholism. Read the book,
Tough Love, by Pauline Neff. Then go for help to a treatment center for
teens and request information on intervention techniques. Intervention,
properly done, works well in most cases. If you saw *The Betty Ford
Story*, you will remember the scene where her family intervened with her.
But it should always be planned and executed with the help of a
professional because intervention is a very powerful technique and can be
dangerous if misapplied.

DEAD END NUMBER 3:

*Other parents and the community often minimize what is going on
with your child or theirs and may work against your efforts.*

Many people still do not recognize alcohol as a drug or alcoholism as
a form of addiction or believe a teenager could really have an incurable
lifetime disease. This myth is widely accepted despite information
available on TV, at schools, in newspapers, the work place, movies,
magazines and books. People would have to live in total isolation from
society not to have the facts available. So why do they not know or
believe the truth? Briefly, the reasons for denial and minimization of the
facts on such a deadly and devastating disease as addiction are:

It is too difficult for some people to accept the truth about
alcoholism's signs, symptoms and results because they may have to
examine their own drinking.

No parents want themselves or their child to be sick. Many families
deny the presence of disease and its symptoms not only in cases of
addiction but with mental illness, epilepsy, multiple sclerosis, and a
myriad of other diseases.

The sense of stigma, shame, or feelings of failure on the part of
parents, schools, and communities will stifle their recognition of the
problem long after it is obvious to others. These entities keep from
'knowing' so they won't have to face the hurt.

It takes time, money, and energy to take action. It is easier to leave attitudes, policies, and laws as they are or let others take care of the problem.

Many parents are stuck in the old patterns of thinking created from misinformation passed on by their parents.

Michelle Smith, another mother from Idaho, tells about dealing with a mother whose daughter was also in trouble with alcohol:

We were thrown together one night at the local hospital. Our daughters Judy and Sheila were in a drunk driving accident. Sheila was driving a man's pickup (an older man who later murdered a woman in our community). They had no business being with this man, who was giving them alcohol and pills. Sheila missed a turn and the pickup rolled three times. My girl, Judy, was thrown and somehow the girls escaped serious injury. Both were really drunk and stoned on pills. They were 15 at the time.

Later, I went with Sheila's mother to their house to discuss what we, as mothers, might do and soon found I could not work with this woman. She told me she gave the girls beer at their home. When I looked shocked, she added, "I know you don't think it's right. But I would rather have them here in front of me, in a controlled place, than out of my sight." This woman totally ignored that most of their drinking was done out of her sight and they were almost killed. She was condoning their drinking by giving beer to them...it was astounding. She also drank a lot—so I think that contributed to her blindness.

The habit of minimizing the consequences of such behavior can be mind-boggling. Parents make statements like:

They're just sowing their oats, being wild or being a kid.

All kids experiment. Do not make a big deal out of it.

It's just a small crowd of druggies; no one pays much attention to them.

There's nothing to do in this community but drink.

A beer bust is traditional, and who wants to destroy all the old traditions?

Natalie B. (now sober in AA) from Edmonds, Washington, recalls growing up in a family of five children with no one in the community alarmed by her family's problem with alcohol and drugs.

My parents didn't believe I or any of my four brothers had a problem with alcohol and drugs. My brothers were always in trouble with the law but when the police came over, my parents just felt my brothers were being ornery and wild. Anytime anything went wrong in the neighborhood, the police showed up at our place. But my parents never considered that alcohol and drugs were the problem.

They took me to counseling because I got pregnant and my Dad wouldn't talk to me. I was thirteen years old. So my Mom arranged for family counseling so we could all live together. But the real issue of alcoholism was never addressed.

No one, neighbors or the school authorities, tried to tell us we had alcohol and drug problems. My parents would not have listened anyway. But looking back, it was obvious that five out of six of us were alcoholic: the parties, the violence (including knife fights), my brothers thefts from me, my parents, each other, and the neighbors.

My father could never admit it because he was an alcoholic himself and if he admitted it in us, he might have to look at himself. My Mom, she just went along with my Dad.

The only way to overcome the habit of minimizing on the part of parents, schools, and communities is to confront the issues. Gain support where you can. Keep a record of all deaths and criminal activity connected with drugs in your community. Give support to any program that helps the cause. Demand that local papers and television stations expose the problems and share the facts as recorded. Do not let other parents say you are overreacting without telling them the facts. Help them face reality by repeatedly presenting these facts. Do not apologize—be determined.

If you cannot see yourself in that role then take care of you and yours. Examine your own drinking and drug use, whether by prescription or just a "social" joint now and then. Is your drug use as harmless as you tell yourself or might there be more to examine? Ask your children. They may just love to tell you what they really think about your drug use and drinking.

Finally, be aware of possible drug abuse by your children from the age of nine until they leave home.

Here is a test that you should periodically go over with your spouse regarding your children. The AWARENESS TEST FOR PARENTS, (Figure 2) is based, in part, on a paper put out by New Beginnings, a chemical dependency treatment program in Denver.

Take this test for each child. Have your spouse take it independent of you. Compare results with your spouse. You will then have a unified awareness test for each child. Ask each other how objective you are in each of your answers.

If *yes* is the answer to four or more of these questions, then there are strong indications that your child may be in trouble with alcohol, marijuana, or other drugs.

If you answer *yes* to a question with an asterisk, you definitely need to seek professional help.

Jean Sable, the Wisconsin activist, says:

Never let anyone tell you that there is nothing you can do about this problem. Each person can educate themselves and make a personal commitment to say 'NO' to chemicals. No one is born knowing everything. With education, problems become challenges. No one wants any person they care about to be drugged, drunk, dependent or dead. Get involved in your school, church, community, service club, or any other place where you can reach people with the truth.

Figure 2.

AWARENESS TEST FOR PARENTS

1. Is your child exhibiting sudden, inappropriate mood changes (irritability, unprovoked hostility or giddiness)?

2. Is your child developing friendships with kids of legal drinking age?

*3. Is your child hanging out with an identified drinking or drug crowd?

4. Is there trouble at school - falling grades, truancy, unexplained absences, especially on Mondays?

5. Is your liquor supply dwindling? What about your pills in the medicine cabinet?

*6. Has anyone (siblings, neighbors, school officials) tried to tell you your child is using drugs or drinking too much?

7. Is your child in trouble with the law?

8. Does your child bad mouth education, television shows, or literature about alcoholism or drug abuse?

*9. Are there signs of medical (ulcers, gastritis, liver inflammation) or emotional problems (depression, overwhelming anxiety, suicidal talk)?

10. Is your child generally dishonest?

11. Do you find obvious signs such as a stash of bottles, beer cans or drug paraphernalia in the bedroom, basement or garage?

12. Do you detect physical signs such as alcohol on the breath, pupil change, redness of eyes, slurred speech or staggering?

13. Does your child smoke cigarettes and/or eat a lot of breath mints?

14. Does your child have flimsy excuses for not being where he said he would be, coming home late, staying out overnight, or getting into trouble at school?

15. Has your child experimented with alcohol and/or drugs or is he spending money on them on a regular basis?

16. Does your child have unproved resentment toward any type of authority figure such as yourself, the police, school officials?

*17. Is your child concerned about his or her use of alcohol or other drugs, including marijuana?

Chapter Highlights

1. Be realistic. Do not expect your teachers, ministers, police, or school board to be the experts on alcoholism and drug abuse. Let the experts be experts. We must not demand that everyone know everything. Do expect them to be aware of the problem and know where and how to refer people.

2. Use the observation sheet (Figure 1) or something like it if you work in the school system. If you are a parent, use the AWARENESS TEST FOR PARENTS. Start doing this from grades four through twelve. Studies show that most kids in recovery began their use and abuse from the ages of nine to eleven, so we need to start observing behaviors at the elementary level.

3. Do not minimize symptoms in your child. Do not let neighbors, friends, relatives, and the law minimize either. If you suspect a problem, you are probably right. Demand that someone help you and help your child.

4. Support laws and programs that support parents and their rights to help and discipline their children.

Resources

Books

Neff, Pauline. *Tough Love (How Parents Can Deal With Drug Abuse)*. Nashville: Abington Press, 1982.

Schaefer, Dick. *Choices & Consequences*. Minneapolis: Johnson Institute Books, 1986.

Videos

Please Remember Me is a one-act play by Jean Sable designed to spark parental awareness about the seriousness of addiction in our children. It is excellent viewing and I recommend it to anyone wishing to raise personal or community awareness. The lines quoted in Chapter 1 and 2 are taken from this play. Jean Sable, 336 S. Whiton, Whitewater, WI 53190 (414) 437-6219.

The Scott Newman Foundation, *Drug Free Kids (A Parent's Guide)* Los Angles: LCA, 1987. A video done by celebrities, this is the best material I have ever viewed on how to react in difficult situations with teenagers. It is straightforward and demonstrates the interactions. It takes a hard line: absolutely NO drug use for any reason.

Chapter 2

The Role of Parents in Treatment and Recovery

Now that you know your child is using, or at least experimenting, what do you do? You may or may not know the seriousness of the problem, but you are certainly concerned. First, stay calm and gather more information. The New Beginnings program in Denver offers some guidelines for parents that are worth following:

Don't threaten, scream, or correct.

Don't accept getting high or drunk as normal.

Don't confront the adolescent when he or she is high or drunk.

Don't blame or make excuses for the person abusing alcohol or drugs.

Don't patronize or condone their abnormal behavior.

Don't give up the ship and accept the adolescent as a loser.

Do talk to the adolescent *only* after the effects of intoxication have worn off.

Do express your concern, love, and willingness to help.

Do allow the adolescent to experience the consequences of his behavior even though these consequences may be painful and/or embarrassing.

Do use community resources to become knowledgeable about alcoholism and chemical dependency.

Do become involved with Families Anonymous and ALANON in your community.

Do seek help from professionals specifically trained in alcoholism and chemical dependency.

There are no hopeless cases. Initial motivation is not a prerequisite. Chances of recovery are better than average with appropriate treatment.

How open-minded or belligerent your child is will influence your decision about whether to include him or her in seeking initial help. You may not want your children to know what you are doing so that you do not frighten them into running away, give them the opportunity to prepare for battle, or talk you out of your concerns or decisions.

Children may try emotional blackmail. They may try to convince us that their abnormal behavior is normal. My daughter tried to convince me that it was normal for teenagers to steal money from their parents, to cut school, to drink, and to disappear for a day or two at a time. She solicited the opinion of an old high school friend of mine, who agreed with my daughter. My friend pointed out to me that I had done many of those same things. But I had to remind her that I was a terrible alcoholic at age fifteen and so using me as an example only showed that it was not normal behavior.

Parents most likely to fall for the "it's normal teenage behavior" story are those who are also Adult Children of Alcoholics (ACOA). One of the main symptoms of ACOAs is that having had no appropriate childhood models, they have to guess what normal is. The best way to deal with this is to attend ACOA meetings and read current books on the subject. You will be amazed how much easier it is to deal with your own children once you recognize dysfunctional patterns.

Another way that teens blackmail their parents is by threatening to hurt themselves, to hate their parents, or to run away. Michelle, the mother in rural Idaho who seemed to be battling the whole town, shares still more of her harassment:

> Things deteriorated so badly after the car accident: stealing, lying, a false pregnancy alarm, disappearing, and possessing cocaine paraphernalia, I simply refused to let Judy go anywhere unchaperoned. Either I, her stepdad, or her friend's parents had to be with her at all times during all activities. And I would not talk on the phone to parents. I had to speak with them in person.
>
> Judy's best friend's parents were very cooperative. They came over often, told me the girls were with them and promised they weren't being left alone. This went on for months. Finally, both girls disappeared after another drunk party at my house when I was in the hospital seeing to my husband's heart attack. I went to Andrea's parents and asked where the girls were. "They told us you had them stay at your place to answer the phone while you were at the hospital.
>
> "Oh hell," her father said, "I'm sick of lying for those girls to you. I'm not going to do it anymore." The mother looked appealingly at me, "I never really lied to you, but I never told you the truth either."
>
> "You mean you lied to me all these months and the girls were doing as they pleased?" Her mother nodded. "Why?" I was appalled. "Because Andrea said she would run away if I didn't lie to you and she means it. I would do anything to keep her here and not worry about her wandering the city streets."

So Andrea's emotional blackmail not only hurt her family but intruded into another mother's attempt to shield her child.

Another form of blackmail is the argument, "You drink with your friends so I'll drink and drug with mine." You raise children, pay taxes, drive, and have all sorts of responsibilities and privileges that your children do not. Your situations are not comparable. This should never be tolerated as a form of logic.

John Travis, an alcoholism counselor from Aurora, Colorado, says:

> What the kid is saying is irrational from a logical standpoint. He's comparing apples to oranges. You have to compare adults to adults and kids to kids. You can't argue because as soon as you say, "You're too young," then they'll ask you to prove it—and how can you prove what too young is? The best minds in history can't. You won't lose this type of no-win argument if you don't play. I suggest to simply say, "You're

not going to drink because it's illegal and I say you're not. And if you do, this is what will happen..."

If logical confrontations turn into illogical arguments, you may need to seek professional help from people trained in the field of chemical dependency. They can help you decide how best to proceed. The amount of involvement by your child in drugs could vary from simple experimentation to blatant drug addiction. And the degree to which they and you are affected will determine the type of help they need.

Examine this scale from the book *Choices & Consequences*, by Dick Schaefer:

FROM USE TO ADDICTION

Use . . . . Learns Mood Swings

Misuse . . . . Seeks Mood Swings

Abuse . . . . Harmfully Involved

Addiction . . . . Harmfully Dependent

Each level requires a different approach and it is important not to misplace your child or saddle him with a label he or she does not deserve.

The first stage simply requires education on the effects and possible results of all drug use. It could call for training in social skills, in explaining how to make choices, in cultivating a positive self-image, and understanding the pitfalls of negative peer pressure.

The second stage may call for a stronger approach, requiring the student to go to some form of counseling or join a school awareness program with positive drug-free peer support. The parents may want to examine their own disciplinary tactics and make sure they are consistent, firm, and clear. They may also, as a family, view televised awareness programs or documentaries for open discussion.

The third stage is more serious and may require all of the suggestions of the first and second stages, plus some form of counseling or required attendance at open meetings of Alcoholics Anonymous (AA), Narcotics

Anonymous (NA), Cocaine Anonymous (CA), or Palmer Drug Abuse Program (PDAP) (see Chapter 9 for definitions).

The issues get complicated with the third and fourth stages. An adolescent who is not suffering from the disease of addiction should not be treated for that disease. Probably only licensed treatment centers will be able to make the distinction between abuse and addiction. But discrimination is required here. The Palmer Drug Abuse Program (PDAP) or its off-shoot programs are designed to deal with abuse. They are also good at spotting someone who needs in-patient treatment and do not hesitate to suggest hospitalization when necessary.

On the other hand, hospital evaluations are not as trustworthy because they are selling a service. Hospital units may justify admissions with the argument: even if the adolescents are not really addicted, it will not hurt them to go through treatment just in case they get the disease some time in the future.

But this argument is not valid. When non-addicted adolescents are mixed with the truly chemically dependent, two things happen. The teens who are not really addicted will not identify with their fellow patients or the content of the treatment. They will pretend to go along with the program until they are discharged from a place they rightfully sense they do not belong. In addition, their attitude and presence will dilute the effectiveness for the young addict who truly needs the treatment.

If the professionals you deal with do not understand the importance of this distinction, you are at the wrong place. *Remember: Good marketing sells bad programs all the time.* Any center must be able to explain to you their evaluation process. It is legitimate to have a ten day in-patient assessment and evaluation process during which they decide what your child's problem really is. One father in Spokane, Washington had admitted his daughter to a Care Unit because of her cocaine use and depression.

> They had her for only two days before they called me back. They had given her a battery of tests, observed her in detox, and interviewed her, then decided she was probably not chemically dependent but needed psychiatric help. I placed her in another institution at that time. But I appreciated their honesty with me. It saved a lot of time and money.

Sometimes treatment center personnel frighten parents into placing their children in centers without the proper screening. This happened to Linda of Idaho Springs, Colorado, who pursued a degree in counseling. I know Linda personally and she is in no way affected by the disease of alcoholism and never was.

> I have been through two treatment programs as an adolescent. One program was for one month, another for thirteen months. My complaints against these programs are that diagnosis was made without much objective information. For one, I was given the MMPI. Because I now have been trained on the proper administration of this test, I can say that this test was not given to me in the proper way. I was given the test at age fourteen with no instructions, no structured setting. Because I did not "respond and admit" to my nonexistent alcoholism, they recommended long-term treatment to my parents. They told them I would die an alcoholic if they didn't leave me in. My parents were scared for my life and ignorant about alcoholism.

Research the treatment center where you place your child. You are dealing with a life-threatening disease—and just as you would want the best cancer specialists, you want the best specialists for the treatment of chemical dependency. Begin your search at your local National Council on Alcoholism or your local Palmer Drug Abuse Program (PDAP). Try asking the parents of any child who has gone for treatment. Or go to ALANON or AA and ask for opinions. The members there have a lot of them. Sober alcoholics are likely to know the centers in your area that do the best job of treating the disease.

After you decide where to go for help, you will probably feel somewhat relieved when some of the pressure is shifted to the professionals. Some parents, out of fear for their child, a lack of knowledge and experience, or other valid reasons, prefer to let the treatment center take over. They defer all decision making to them. It is not necessary to castigate yourself for this. It is your choice. If your child had cancer, you may or may not choose to become an expert on cancer. You would turn your child over to the oncologist, follow his or her advice, see that your child gets all the required care, and leave the rest to God or whatever your personal belief system says.

This is your child's disease, not yours. *You did not cause it and you cannot make him or her well.* You do not have that power no matter who suggests you might. Once your adolescent is safely on the way to treatment, you have five main responsibilities.

Offer love and support and have realistic expectations

By doing everything necessary to place your child in treatment, you are already showing your love. It is not necessary to tell you, "Love your kid." Even by reading this book, you are showing extraordinary love and caring.

Many parents forget quickly that their children have a very serious life-threatening disease. I recall the first and only aftercare parents' group I attended. I had been excited about attending and maybe gaining insights into how other parents were coping with alcoholism/addiction in their kids. We sat at a long table and each parent spoke of how the week had gone. One mother said she was glad her daughter had made the bed and even though she had a few beers she spoke nicely to her grandmother so she figured progress had been made.

A father said he locked his son out of the house during the day so he would not steal his booze and was angry that his son had not found a job. Another parent said their daughter had not argued or bad-mouthed them in a week and they felt good about the changing attitude. Yet another parent discussed the fact that her kid went to a rock concert with another graduate from the treatment center and was frightened they had used drugs together.

It went on like that with parents discussing if their children's attitudes had changed and whether they had cleaned their rooms. No one spoke of the sickness, the horrible disease that was killing their kids. Not one child had stayed clean and sober. No one mentioned getting their kids to AA, or working a program of sobriety, or sponsors, or anything to do with recovery from the alcoholism. I felt they had all somehow missed the point. I never went back.

If we, as parents, expect treatment to make our children stop swearing, stop smoking, dress more conservatively or clean up their room, then we are searching for the wrong result. Our teen is suffering from a disease, a serious disease—the single leading cause of death in teenagers—the third leading cause of death in adults.

After treatment, do not fret over their behavior problems and the things that annoy you. Focus on recovery from the disease. Encourage them to attend Twelve Step meetings and aftercare groups (one everyday is good for the first year). If they are hanging out with their old drug friends, take action again. But if the teen has a sponsor and is maintaining contact, the process of sobriety is probably working.

The addicted teen is fighting for his or her life. This is not a test. And if our son or daughter can possibly stay in a Twelve Step program, we are batting 100 percent over the majority of teens that are coming out of treatment. Do not worry about the obnoxious teenage behavior displayed today but be concerned about them working a drug-free program. If they stay clean and sober long enough, the obnoxious behavior will eventually go away.

Know that addiction is a disease and don't treat it like anything else

No matter what you have heard or read, the latest research on the subject has concluded that addiction is a disease. There was a time when some medical literature made ridiculous statements. I was twenty-one years old, in my first year of sobriety when a nurse in a Canadian clinic handed me a pamphlet that read, "If you do sports like tennis, you will not get VD." There was a time when the Red Cross and other medical experts recommended butter for burns. There was a time when epilepsy was considered possession by evil spirits. We grow up. We gain knowledge. Experience is a great teacher.

Alcoholism and any other drug addiction are diseases. Addiction is not a question of being weak-willed; it is not a mental problem; it is not a behavioral problem; it is not a moral problem; it is not a problem of the poor. It is a disease, a malfunctioning of the body for a variety of reasons.

If you have any flicker of a doubt left regarding this, do two things. First, read the chapter "Disease or Habit" in this book. Second, go to your library and look up the latest medical research on the topic. Only two or three studies should be necessary but they will convince you that chemical addiction is a biological phenomenon sometimes genetic and always medically verifiable (see examples, Resources).

Make an informed decision about the level of involvement you will take in your child's treatment and aftercare

Each family situation is different and the decision about how much to participate in treatment and recovery will depend on many factors. Your economic situation may influence the decision as may other family concerns. Whether or not you are a single parent will affect your decision. The age of the child is also a factor. Obviously, if your child is twelve, he or she will be under your care for a long time. You may want to learn more and participate more fully than the parent whose child is eighteen or nineteen and ready to leave home.

Make an informed decision and do not let others, especially professionals, badger you into guilt for not doing things their way. Although the parent may be as involved in treatment of his child's addiction as if it was treatment of another severe illness, it is not necessary to learn everything about addiction. Do not accept unwarranted guilt for the situation, nor do you have to join a myriad of programs. The whole world does not have to revolve around one child, unless you want it to.

Make sure you are not an enabler.

It could kill your child. Refusing to be an enabler means giving responsibility for the addiction to the only person who can do something about the drug use: your addicted or drug abusing teen. The child will be more likely to assume responsibility if you do not shield him or her from the consequences of drug abuse.

Practice Tough Love, which means simple things like not writing excuses to school when there are none. Do not bail your child out of jail, pay book fines, make excuses to authorities, or buy concert tickets. Reading the book, *Tough Love*, or attending the meetings of ALANON, Co-Dependents Anonymous, Families Anonymous, Narcanon, or ACOA will help you understand and implement Tough Love. Any one of these groups can help you see the value and learn the techniques of letting the addict be responsible for his or her own actions.

The outline on the next page may also help you.

ENABLING BEHAVIORS OUTLINE

1. Denying: "My kid does not have a problem."

   Results in:

   Expecting the chemical dependent teen to be rational.

   Expecting the chemical dependent teen to stop because you said so.

   Accepting blame.

2. Drinking and smoking dope with the adolescent to "teach them how."

3. Justifying their drugging by agreeing with their rationalizations:

   "All the kids go to keggers."

   "I'd be a nerd if I didn't."

4. Ignoring the problem because "They'll grow out of it."

5. Minimizing:

   "It's not so bad."

   "Things will get better when...."

   "All kids test their wings."

6. Protecting your child from legal, social and school consequences by:

   Bailing them out.

   Writing excuses to cover up.

   Giving them money when they don't deserve it.

   Looking the other way when your own money disappears.

7. Avoiding the situation by soothing feelings with tranquilizers, food or work.

8. Lecturing by blaming and criticizing.

9. Taking over their responsibilities by:

   Letting them slide on their chores

   Giving them the car to drive when they haven't earned it

10. Feeling superior: telling them what it was like when you were a kid.

11. Controlling: "You're grounded until you're thirty."

12. Waiting: "God will take care of it."

(Based on the work of Harriet Davis and adapted to adolescents, New Beginnings, Denver.)

Take care of yourself

You are a very important person. You have done the very best you could. Do not blame yourself for your child's addiction. Do not let others blame you either. If you do not find peace and happiness within yourself, no one will find it for you. Ultimately, your child will have to arrest his or her own disease: No one is going to take care of you—but you.

Chapter Highlights

1. Do not let your kids use emotional blackmail on you and convince you their abnormal behavior is normal. Do not allow them to threaten you or draw you into illogical arguments.

2. Remember that good marketing sells bad programs.

3. Beware of numerous things in your search for a recovery program. Just as you would research a new physician or dentist, research the treatment centers.

4. Understand that addiction is a disease, not a bad habit, moral problem, weakness of will, or psychological problem.

5. Make your own decision about how involved you want to become in your child's treatment. Do not let others pressure you into doing it their way. They do not live in your family and are not equipped to make those decisions.

6. Avoid enabling. To cover up or pick up for your child is not being fair to yourself nor will it help your son or daughter to recover. Do attend some ALANON, Narcanon, Co-Dependents Anonymous, Families Anonymous, or Adult Children of Alcoholic meetings to learn helpful techniques. You may want to send your other children to Alateen or attend the Palmer Drug Abuse Program as a family.

Resources

Books

Schaefer, Dick. *Choices & Consequences*, Minneapolis: Johnson Institute, 1988.

Baron, J. *The Parent Handbook of Drug Abuse and Treatment*, DAPA, PO Box 741329, Houston, TX 77274-1329

Neff, Pauline. *Tough Love (How Parents Can Deal With Drug Abuse)*, Nashville: Abingdon Press, 1982.

The International Classification of Diseases, Fourth Edition. (1991). Diseases Tabular List (DHHS) Publication No. (PHS) 91-1260. Washington, D.C.: U. S. Government Printing Office.

Periodicals

Rinaldi, R. C., E. M. Steindler, B. B. Wilford, D. Goodwin. 1988. "Clarification and Standardization of Substance Abuse Terminology." *JAMA* 259: 555-557.

Chapter 3
Codependency Cop-out

The trend in the field of treating teenage alcoholics is to interview the entire family and examine what part members play in relation to the addict. Some methods of systemic analysis categorize everyone in the family as ill and in need of treatment. Systemic analysis has somehow shifted from examining family dynamics and making appropriate recommendations to focusing on individuals' dysfunctional roles.

Some institutions define codependency as a disease entity. Treatment centers usually describe codependency as particular patterns of behavior found in most members of chemically dependent families.

There are problems with seeing everyone surrounding an addict as somehow *sick* and *dysfunctional*. We should not diagnosis as sick spouses or parents who, out of limited knowledge, love, or religious conviction, have enabled or coerced an addict they love. A more useful example of sick is a father who bails his son out of jail repeatedly, refusing to accept victim reports that he is a rapist, or the wife who remains with her husband who drinks, beats her, loses jobs, blames her and after ten miserable years still cries in a weak voice, "but I love him." Sick is the father who has molested his daughter since childhood and now refuses to go to counseling because he believes his daughter liked it.

A father who bails his son out of jail more than once, tries desperately to "talk some sense into the boy," who tries to teach his son how to drink responsibly, then beats the boy up after finding marijuana in his car and hearing his son say "Fuck you" is not a sick codependent. He and these other spouses and parents have not been trained to deal with addicts. They need information and skills, not individual psychotherapy. It is not useful to treat him for some elusive disease. It is the job of the professional to teach these skills to those close to the addict.

Ruby, a mother from Tri-cities, Washington, shares her problems about her nineteen year old daughter:

> I allowed my daughter to move home because she lost her live-in and needed to get her feet on the ground. I found myself babysitting Tyrone, my grandbaby, while she partied all weekend. Then I had to baby-sit him while she nursed a hangover. Then we got into screaming matches about her not being a good mother to Tyrone. I didn't know what to do. I was at my wit's end.

These are not the words of a sick codependent enabler but of a loving, concerned, uninformed woman who needs to be informed and taught how to detach herself while protecting her grandchild.

Use discretion with ACOA and codependency issues

With adolescents, it is important to not imply that they are addicts/alcoholics because of a dysfunctional family. That message undermines attempts to arrest the disease. It gives the young adult:

> a) a ready made excuse to shift responsibility for his behavior, "It's not my responsibility to stop this behavior—it's the whole family's."

> b) a way to make fault-finding and blaming a block to recovery, "This isn't my fault in the first place so I needn't struggle to change."

> c) an excuse by insinuating that this isn't *really* a disease but a family systems problem. This leaves the impression that if the system changes, the addiction will go away.

> d) a reason to feel relatively incompetent to handle present circumstances, to alter his or her world and effect change. They can feel that they are at the mercy of conditions in the family over which they have no control.

Consider the following from *Adult Children Of Alcoholics*, by Janet Woititz:

> Disruption is not exclusive to the alcoholic family system. So-called "normal" families have their share of ups and downs as well. Children living in "normal" families can have behavior problems and be disruptive. Some of this is part of growing up and some of it may mean more serious difficulties. The key is to know the differences, and in the family complicated by alcohol, it is harder to sift things out realistically.

Adult Children Of Alcoholics proposes a conceptual framework for explaining certain features of the lives of ACOAs. Woititz's message is about knowledge—self-knowledge and insight into our dysfunctional families. These insights help us make healthy choices. Her message is about knowledge, choice and action.

Professionals and non-professionals alike use Dr. Woititz's concepts to explain sickness in our society. If teen addicts abdicate responsibility for their behavior because Mom was an alcoholic and Mom's grandad was an alcoholic, Dr. Woititz says, "They've missed the point."

Teen addicts already try to blame schools, parents, siblings, and legal systems for everything they do. They do not need additional excuses using ACOA and codependency material out of context.

Yet it is being done all the time. Treatment center staff are reluctant to examine their programs. It is much easier for a therapist to get Johnny to admit he has low self-esteem because Mom was drunk in his formative years than to get Johnny to admit he has choices of his own or to get him to admit he has an incurable disease that may kill him.

Tragically, many treatment programs are allowing the belief, either by commission or omission, that dysfunctional families cause alcoholism in the adolescent. Dysfunctional families may increase or hasten the manifestation of addictive behavior but they don't cause the genetic proclivity or brain chemistry components of the disease (see Chapter 4, Disease or Habit).

Neither do families cause diabetes. But consider: unhealthy lifestyles along with gross eating habits may contribute to the age of onset. If a family has a history of aggressive diabetes then there is a good chance that one or more of their offspring will have it. A healthy family will work together to educate their children, get regular check-ups and practice prevention. When a child shows the beginning signs of illness (known as borderline diabetes), a stricter form of prevention ensues: eliminating simple carbohydrates in the diet, proper eye care, attention to sores, etc. In an unhealthy family dysfunctional members may ignore symptoms, avoid preventive steps, and not seek medical monitoring. When initial problems begin, they exert feeble attempts to control the disease, but employ no specific course of action. That is a family that is contributing to the disease. If the diabetes escalates to life threatening proportions and the child will not take his insulin or insists on ten colas a day (which happens), hospitalization or other professional help may become necessary.

Pursuing the analogy, it is detrimental to recovery to have professionals telling the patient it is not his or her fault that he or she drinks ten colas a day. The fact that the patient's dysfunctional family is contributing to his or her low self-esteem, lack of control, difficulty with authority and relationship troubles is irrelevant. They did not cause the diabetes and they will not cure it. Again, this is not to say that knowledge about dysfunctional families is not helpful in treating addiction, but it should be introduced in proper perspective. The fact is there are some basically healthy families with some very sick children.

Many addicts don't come from dysfunctional and codependent families

Mrs. Smith from Idaho finally was able to place her daughter in treatment:

> I remember the intake nurse insisting I go to ALANON and that I had to have real problems because Judy was alcoholic. I didn't happen to agree with her. I had eighteen years sobriety myself; the nurse didn't know anything about our family.

> I remember seeing another man in there who was also being told he needed to change his behavior toward his daughter and his family. He had fifteen years sobriety and I saw him putting Crystal into treatment as healthy and all his interactions with her as pretty normal.

> One night in a parents' therapy group all the families gathered in a circle to say something supportive to a graduating patient. Everyone said sweet things except the father. The father told his son, "I don't believe you've heard a thing they've told you in here. I give you one day." The boy smiled and looked down at his shoes.

The counselor and I exchanged glances. That was an example of a dysfunctional family: a father who blasts the son on what should have been a happy occasion and a son who smiles in response.

I shared the incident with a friend, RaNae (sober six years and having raised six kids). I told her how the father displayed his own sickness.

"Not necessarily," she commented. "You're talking about a father who is at his rope's end. Can you imagine what he's been through to drive him to the point of admitting his son to treatment? Remember what your daughter has put you through. Maybe he knows his son better then all of you."

And in the end, he did know. His son went out and began using again in several weeks.

None of us can judge whether or not the father and son in this story were part of a dysfunctional family. But this father's (or any parent's) utter frustration and deep anger should not be used as a sign of family dysfunction. Intensive evaluations of the family are needed to conclude that the family is dysfunctional or falls into the ACOA or codependency category.

The word of the adolescent is not enough to evaluate a family

Teenagers often feel like victims as a normal course of development. They go through a stage of blaming parents for life's inadequacies and find fault in all areas. This tendency becomes deceptive when coupled with the addict's lack of honesty. Another mother shared with me:

My daughter played the victim role to the highest degree. She spoke of child abuse with her counselors like she was beat half to death on a weekly basis. When in fact I "abused" her maybe ten to fifteen times until she was eleven. There was never any blood or bruises and I went for help and got it. From the ages of eleven to seventeen she only got two whippings and one was because she attacked me first.

The concept of other family members being sick along with the addict began years ago with ALANON

From the concept for ALANON (an organization for the spouse of an alcoholic who is drawn into the disease) grew the concept "codependency" (the idea that a spouse, employer, parent, or sibling enables the alcoholic/addict through certain behavior). "Adult children of alcoholics" are children affected in some measure by an alcoholic/addicted parent. Now ACOA in its broadest sense covers all members of dysfunctional families.

In AA, they used to say that a "normal" woman or man might mistakenly marry an alcoholic, but would not stay married to him or her once the abuse, economic problems, irrationality, and dishonesty became apparent and chronic. Anyone who did stick around was obviously "sick" to some degree. Members of AA described that as unhealthy behavior or "ALANON" behavior. AA members used this concept to justify urging other members to seek help for their unhealthy marriages.

Now professionals and many misinformed lay people who support ALANON and ACOA try to apply this concept to all families—Any family who has an alcoholic member is affected by alcoholism; therefore, any family with an alcoholic is sick.

Not true. Parents do not choose to have alcoholic kids; and in my opinion taking their kids to treatment is a healthy parental response. It may have come at the end of a long series of maneuvers to help their child, all of which failed, but the family is succeeding if they are seeking help and still working toward growth.

What old-timers in AA used to observe in an ALANON woman or man cannot be applied to the family of the teenage addict. The parents did not "choose" to stay related to their kid as the ALANON spouses chose to stay married to an alcoholic for twenty-five years. Parents are dealing with one, two, or three years of addiction as opposed to ten, twenty, or thirty years. The same patterns of denial and enabling have not always developed.

Professionals in chemical dependency need to be cognizant of the history behind the CoDA (Co-Dependents Anonymous) and ACOA issues so they can judge the validity of their center's emphasis on them. Chemical dependency counselors may want to ask themselves these important questions:

> Can misconceptions about and mistreatment of alcoholism/ addiction be eliminated in members of the addict's family without insisting every member join a program to get help?

Can we get an honest evaluation of the family dynamics by relying solely on the chemically dependent child's testimony?

Are we using CoDA and ACOA to supplement an inadequate treatment agenda and shift attention from recovery of the addict to recovery of an ill-defined disease in the family? Do we find sickness in everyone?

Finally, examine the chart of Adolescent Addiction and Parental Reaction (Figure 3). There is a natural progression in family dynamics in reaction to the sick member. It takes a little education and some self-assertion before most parents can stop "reacting" in inappropriate ways.

Figure 3.

ADOLESCENT ADDICTION AND PARENTAL REACTION
EARLY STAGES

Addict	Parent
Begins smoking marijuana	Awareness of Problem:
Sneaking and stealing booze	Money
Blackouts	School
Overuses medications	Chores
Heavy experimentation with drugs	Attitude
Urgent requests for money	Appearance
Preoccupation with drugs	Nagging starts
Lies to cover use	The need to "control" increases
Hangs out with drug crowd	Suspects friends are bad influence
Hides most of this from parents	**Begins to deny and rationalize**

MIDDLE STAGES

Addict	Parent
Abusive or mocking attitude toward non-users	Begins to cover-up for teen's behavior
Tries to limit use	Extracts promises
Changes drugs to control use	Guilt about parenting
Alibiing	Blames child's friends
Drastic mood swings	Begins to threaten
Relief using	Escalates discipline
Emotional withdrawal	Emotional withdrawal
Probable promiscuity	Begin:
May start dealing to support use	Headaches
Drops out of school or school activities	Ulcers
Cannot hide troubles	Nerves
	May increase own drug use
	May seek help

ADVANCED OR CHRONIC

Addict	Parent
Weekend binges or daily using	Assumes blame for bad parenting
Unknown fears	Self-respect slips as influence on child slips
Physical symptoms common to drug of choice	Overreactive attempts to discipline
Gives up on controlling use	Retaliation:
Irrationality regarding school, friends, money, family, authority	Calls police
Has to deal, steal, and con to acquire drugs	Kicks kid out and recants
Chronic problem in family	May start physical or verbal abuse
Physical withdrawal	Neglects other family members
Addiction no longer hidden	**Sincere search for help**

Addiction in the adolescent is a primary disease, in the medical biological sense.

Addiction is not a family disease unless every member of the family has it.
   Professionals should stop calling it a family disease.
   It adds to or creates a family discomfort and dysfunction.

MS, thyroid disease, and schizophrenia create similar situations where family members first react to initial symptoms; then act in seeking help; then adapt to recovery. In these situations, one family member's disease affects the entire family structure.

The professional's job is to help the family cope, not cure them of something they do not have.

Chapter Highlights

1. Use discretion with ACOA and CoDA issues in adolescent treatment. It is easy to give adolescents excuses to shift responsibility for their behavior to the family and to feel that they are at the mercy of their family's "original sin," over which they have no control.

2. Insinuating that a family has an underlying systemic problem gives the impression that alcoholism is not actually a disease and that if the family problem is treated, the alcoholism/addiction will go away.

3. Remember, parents do not choose to have addicted children. Some basically healthy families can have sick children.

Resources

Books

Cermak, T.L. *Diagnosing and Treating Co-dependence*. Minneapolis: Johnson Institute Books, 1986.

Woititz, Janet. *Adult Children of Alcoholics*. Pompano Beach: Health Communications, Inc., 1983.

Chapter 4
Disease or Habit

The American Medical Association has given formal recognition to the disease concept of alcoholism since 1956. Recognizing alcohol and other drug dependency as an illness involves several things:

The illness can be described.

The course of the illness is predictable and progressive.

The disease is primary—that is, it is not just a symptom of some other underlying disorder.

It is permanent.

It is terminal. If left untreated, it inevitably results in premature death.

The professional may be saying now, "I know this." Yet:

4.6 million teens are in trouble with alcohol.

The average age of initial use is between nine and eleven.

Alcoholism is probably in part genetic. Alcoholism and addiction are a bio\psycho\social diseases.

The disease of addiction does not respect age.

However some professionals do not believe what they know.

The biggest single obstacle in the recovery of teenage alcoholics is the fact that too many professionals do not believe the adolescent is that sick. It's hard to convince someone that they really do not believe teenagers can be full-blown alcoholic/addicts. Even though therapists, directors and older sponsors in AA and NA pay lip service to such words, their actions contradict the message.

In a recent study Dr. Michael Marshall and I compared the attitudes of counselors on adolescent-only units to counselors on units that treat both adolescents and adults. We found that counselors in adolescent-only centers impose more parental control (dress codes, behavior control, food and beverage restrictions) than counselors on the combined units. One might be tempted to say, "of course the counselors respond to their teenage clients with a parental attitude. They're dealing with kids." But on combined units or adult units, adolescents and adults are treated the same (see Appendix 1). If adolescent-only counselors believe that adolescents have the same serious disease as adults, why is their treatment attitude different?

A closer look at treatment programs reveals that staff frequently and repeatedly react to teenage patients in the following ways.

They call a chronic, devastating primary disease a habit.

They tell patients that relapse is part of recovery.

They refuse patients cookies and coffee as a part of recovery.

They teach that if the patient learns not to swear, wear jeans with holes, hang heavy metal posters, their recovery chances will improve.

Treatment centers throughout the country do just these things in the name of recovery (each will be examined in detail in Chapter 5: The Structure of Treatment). Imagine an adult unit that did the above. A program developer from Aurora, CO, Linda Yoakem, shares:

> It seems that there are really two programs and two diseases in the minds of many treatment programs: there is a "kiddie" program for those with "no real problem" or "kiddie alcoholism." When you get older, then you get the "real" disease, the "adult alcoholism." It's almost as though adolescents are expected to get a different disease when they get older.

I requested to sit in on some adolescent aftercare groups in a center in Denver as part of my research for this book. The director and I discussed philosophy and we concurred that alcoholism is a disease. I picked up the hospital packet (one given to incoming patients) to familiarize myself with policies and procedures.

This hospital's brochure on chemical dependency had a separate section for adolescents in which they referred to treatment as "stopping a drug habit." A forty-five day intensive medical program is not needed to treat a "habit."

That same brochure reads, "Because alcoholism is a chronic and progressive disease, adolescents who drink have a much higher potential than their non-drinking peers for developing alcohol-related problems." However, adolescent alcoholics/addicts are not being treated as having serious problems.

The brochure goes on to describe adult alcoholism as a disease recognized by the AMA and characterized as "drinking of alcohol (that) turns into a health-destroying physical and mental compulsion." So it appears that adult alcoholism is treated as a real disease but adolescent alcoholism is not. Probably we harbor prejudices that we do not acknowledge.

Our buried prejudices stem from many areas. Our parents taught us that alcohol was just a social drink that made one feel good. It is hard to dispel parental messages regardless of what we now know. Society taught us that alcoholics were old men stumbling around skid row drinking wine. It is hard to dispel societal messages regardless of what we now know. Gambling, sex, and shoplifting are now being described as diseases casting doubt on the real biological dimensions of addiction. There is a common belief that adolescents have not had time to develop the disease even though time is not always a factor.

Teenage alcoholism is not:

A special disease

A special stage of the disease

Pre-disease

My own situation reflects this:

My mother drank and used drugs from ages sixteen to thirty-eight. In that time, she abused her children, lost an opportunity for a college education, went from job to job, marriage to marriage, and humiliated herself as the town drunk in a California mountain community.

I drank and did drugs from ages fifteen to twenty-one, became a stripper to support my booze and speed habits, made money off of getting girls to pose nude for men, and slept with anyone who would supply me.

My daughter began her drug and drinking career at thirteen years old. At eighteen she is very ill and still using. Death sometimes seems preferable to this state. Addictive disease is no respecter of age and its seriousness does not necessarily increase with age.

There is no distinction between "adult addiction" and "kiddie addiction." Parents, professionals, and the addicted teenagers themselves have to understand the biological as well as the psychological and spiritual components of addiction. Everyone is an expert when it comes to talking about drinking and drugs. And a lot of people use words that mean one thing to them, but quite another to someone else. For purposes of simplicity, when speaking of the disease, the words alcoholic, addict, chemically dependent, pill head, pot head, and other terms referring to an addicted person will be used interchangeably. They refer to the same thing, the Addictions Syndrome.

What we see in young people who are hooked on a chemical is a physical compulsion, a mental obsession, and a lack of spirituality—call it self-centeredness. The disease is marked by a compulsive use of substances, powerlessness over what they do, an impairment of the normal state of health that interferes with our thrust for life and joy in living—all disguised as "better living through chemistry."

Most therapists and other treatment personnel have no trouble working with the psychological aspects of the Addictions Syndrome. Traditionally, professionals have categorized it as a mental problem. The spiritual aspect is usually addressed in the Twelve Step program or a person's religious associations. It is the biological component that seems to present the major barrier in general acceptance of the disease concept—especially in adolescents.

Any good treatment center should and will have information about the effects of alcoholism: the addict's preoccupation with mind altering chemicals, how addicts adapt their lifestyles to facilitate use of chemicals, about faulty memory, chemical blackouts, and euphoric recall. But few offer materials that explain the physiology of alcoholism.

Professionals should take inventory of their knowledge of chemical dependency and ask themselves—Do I really believe what I know?

There are two main types of disease:
   a) infectious (the kind you catch from others) and
   b) functional (when the system malfunctions negatively affecting the body).

Alcoholism is a functional disease. A purely biological definition of chemical dependency describes alcoholism and other addictions as a neuro-transmitter deficiency in the brain coupled with other bodily malfunctions.

Scientists know that there are brain wave deficits in alcoholics. The P-3 brain wave response to certain stimuli is absent in some children of alcoholics, in practicing alcoholics and in long-time sober alcoholics. These deficits can be used as a biological marker for those of us in the field. There are also blood tests which show that two enzymes found in blood platelets react differently in alcoholics and non-alcoholics. These tests can identify about 75 percent of those at risk for alcoholism. Science is now catching up to what alcoholics have long suspected—alcoholism is a biological disease.

As long as we believe in the biological component of addiction, we will never again think of age as a factor in its development. We will never regard teenage alcoholics as "potential" alcoholics, that were "caught in time," that can be taught "responsible choices in using chemicals," or that they may "someday outgrow" their addiction.

Chemical dependency is a chronic and progressive illness. It continues to get worse. The bottom line is insanity or death.

I know this, but do I believe it? Any professional who believes this will never make light of relapse in the adolescent. Many therapists and counselors urge their patients not to be ashamed if they use again after treatment. In fact, relapse is so common that it is often described as a part of recovery.

Relapse is an indicator of disease—but is it part of recovery? *People die, kill others, become disabled, brain-damaged, cause birth defects in unborn children and go to jail in relapse.*

It is not a part of recovery. Yes, teach teenagers to return to recovery, but teach them to return because of the seriousness of relapse, not because it is "no big deal."

Chemical dependency tends to create and magnify emotional problems. Chemical dependency is not caused by bad parents, nagging wives, guilt and debts, nor is it caused by bad nerves, a weak character or lack of self-control.

I know this but do I believe it? If you really believe this you will not confuse CoDA or ACOA issues with the recovery of your patient. You will never let them believe that if their parents straighten up, they will no longer have the need to use. You will never allow them to shift responsibility for their behavior or disease to their parents, siblings, schools, courts, race, or even poor self image or economic background. Such factors may explain why they pick up that first fix, snort, pill, or drink but they never cause the disease.

Chemical dependency is treatable. It cannot be cured. The only way to stop the progression of the illness is to abstain from mood-altering chemicals. Because the illness does not go away, we refer to addicts as "recovering," not "recovered."

I know this but do I believe it? Addiction is treatable by abstaining only. We put people into treatment so they can withdraw safely, get them away from the mind-altering chemical long enough to make a rational decision, teach them about their disease, and get them on a program that will help them live without relying on chemicals. In reality, they treat themselves—treatment gives them the opportunity to learn how to abstain for a lifetime. It interrupts the cycle of the disease in a safe and instructional atmosphere and provides professionals the opportunity to instill motivation. Generally practitioners who believe they can "treat" or affect cure are those that still treat addiction as psychological and familial only, not recognizing the biological aspects of the syndrome.

Chemical dependency can be inherited, or the system can be chemically abused for so long that it "breaks down." I know this but do I believe it? Cancer can strike children or adults. The same thing applies to addiction. Some people are born alcoholic/addictive and manifest the disease from the first drink, just as some are born with heart trouble or epilepsy. Some people are born with a predisposition to addiction which will become apparent after they abuse chemicals for a certain length of time.

And some people will abuse chemicals to the point of addiction or what appears to be addiction, but not really have the Addictions Syndrome as we know it. Once the chemical is out of their system, they do not have the compulsion or obsession that alcoholics and other chemical dependents have. Studies of Vietnam veterans proved that some people can use drugs addictively, but not have the disease that is, they stop when drugs are no longer useful to them. Many soldiers were addicted in Vietnam and astounded scientists when they returned to the states and stopped using. The big crisis in addiction that was predicted simply failed to appear. About the same percentage of veterans continued their addiction upon returning as would have started had they stayed home, about one in ten.

More than one disease is used here to illustrate the similarities in functional and genetically predisposed diseases. The disease state is dominant. If you have the disease, you are no longer predisposed to it nor will stopping the high risk behaviors cure it, although it may help arrest or control the symptoms.

For example in High Risk Behavior number one, if someone smokes but is not genetically predisposed to weak lungs, he may pound himself with smoking for thirty years and only have an annoying cough to show for it. On the other hand, if his father had emphysema, his chances of developing the disease increase. If he engages in other high risk behaviors such as living in a polluted city, his chances of getting lung disease (and getting it earlier) increase. If he works in a coal mine, his chances increase even more.

Engaging in high risk behavior does not always mean a person will succumb to disease. Not everyone who smokes or works in a coal mine gets emphysema. The analogy can continue with each example of predisposition and high risk behavior. How much hammering each person can take before going into the disease state is determined by genetic

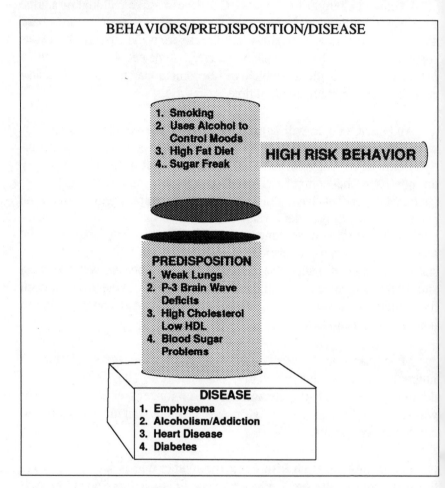

structure and external factors. This is an important distinction when it comes to intake evaluation and treatment (discussed more fully in Chapter 5, The Structure of Treatment).

It is vitally important that every professional in the field of addiction be an expert on the disease.

We must know what the disease is and how to diagnose it.

We must know what it is not.

This is our field and people's lives depend on our studying the research, participating in research, and continuing to learn.

Chapter Highlights

1. Some professionals do not believe what they know about addiction and continue to treat adolescent addiction as something less serious than adult addiction.

2. Teen alcoholism is not a special disease, a special stage of the disease, or a pre-disease phase.

3. Each one of us professionals must inventory our own hidden prejudices about chemical dependency. We are responsible for the subtle messages that slip through to our patients and our patients' families.

4. Each one of us in this field must be an expert on what this disease is and what it is not. We are responsible for keeping up on the latest research and continuing our education.

Resources

Books

Diagnostic and Statistical Manual of Mental Disorders. Washington DC: American Psychiatric Association, 1987.

Marshall, Shelly. *Young, Sober & Free,* Center City, Mn: Hazelden, 1978.

Research

Nehr, T. 1991. Altered States. *Professional Counselor* 5: 31-35.

Tabakoff, B., et al. 1988. Alcoholism: A New and Promising Blood Test. *New England Journal of Medicine* 318: 134.

Videos

George Page, *Mind/Addiction* (volume 4) 1988. WNET/New York: Educational Broadcasting Corporation.

Section II

Developing Treatment That Works

Introduction

We are all working together to help adolescent addicts and their families recover. But we are in the infancy stages of program development for adolescent treatment. As we explore many avenues, we discover paths that help and paths that hinder.

Traveling this country from California to North Carolina, visiting treatment programs, I have interviewed directors, physicians, therapists, and adolescents in and out of recovery. I have observed strategies that worked and those that did not. Some programs are better than others. All programs have some value and none are so good that there is nothing left to improve. Our current adolescent centers have a recovery rate of less then 5 percent (see Appendix 2). Each one of these centers can raise that success rate.

The chapters in this section challenge some attitudes and assumptions from the past and present ideas for improving many areas of adolescent treatment. Professionals in the field are better equipped than any other group of people to make meaningful changes in addictions treatment.

Chapter 5, The Structure of Treatment, discusses the inherent problems of assessing the disease and treating addiction. Chapter 6, The

Content of Treatment, examines outcome expectations and propose realistic goals. Chapter 7, Skills of the Staff, explores specific procedures for dealing with young people.

Chapter 5

The Structure of Treatment

People in the Palmer Drug Abuse Program, Alcoholics Anonymous, Narcotics Anonymous and Cocaine Anonymous all believe that young people who are addicted can and do get straight. But a less than 5 percent success rate seems to contradict this belief. We are just now beginning to identify what makes a strong program. We are in the process of searching for the best program, the perfect program.

The perfect program, of course, does not exist. Anyone searching for final answers is not going to find them. But those searching for better answers will find them, as programs are tested and improved to help the teenage addict/alcoholic. Since addiction treatment research is in its infancy, we must expect that some methods now in use will not prove to be effective. We must be prepared to assess and change ineffective treatment strategies.

Most adolescent treatment now takes place in for-profit incorporated centers. The corporations dictate policies and procedures in an attempt to create a uniform treatment environment in all their branches. These centers, with their plush interiors and credentialed personnel, impress parents, courts, and psychiatrists. Their rules and methods appear sound. But appearances have nothing to do with success.

·

Professionals fail more often than they succeed in treatment and the economics of addiction treatment reflect these failures. Insurance companies are questioning the thousands of dollars reimbursed to hospitals having a less then 5 percent success with teens. Parents are questioning treatment efficacy, and now the professionals working with teens are questioning the present methods.

How is treatment structured? In this chapter, we will examine three areas: 1) intake, detox and evaluation, 2) rules and regulations, 3) mainstreaming adolescents.

Intake, Detox and Evaluation

Treatment begins with intervention and intake techniques. The first thing to be determined is whether the patient needs in-patient or out-patient treatment. A myriad of variables must be considered: the degree of chemical dependency, motivation of the patient and even insurance coverage. If they have no insurance coverage, patients may have to be referred to or put in a charity bed. They may be able to afford out-patient but not in-patient treatment. In-patient treatment is required if the patient is very ill during withdrawal, and desirable if the patient lacks motivation.

Most centers have a three to ten day detoxification and assessment period in which they make some very important decisions regarding the adolescent. Regardless of the cause of the teenager's abuse of drugs, the clinician must first determine whether the patient requires in-patient treatment or could be referred to other programs.

Thus teens who suffer from a disease are separated from teens manifesting behavior problems that drive families and society crazy. If you have a "behavioral problem" adolescent misusing drugs or a teen manifesting delinquency, mental, or socialization problems, it is important not to combine the "behavioral problem" teen with the addicts. If you do, you cannot effectively treat both. Treating teens with behavior problems who misuse or abuse drugs is not drug treatment, it is prevention. If a child has a psychiatric problem, he or she needs a psychiatric ward. Prevention of addiction and psychiatric care are entirely different from treating the incurable and chronic disease of addiction.

When the various problem groups are combined, treatment for each is diluted and not as effective.

Prevention belongs in the realm of education, drug-free support groups, and self-esteem motivators (Remember, I am speaking of preventing drug misuse and abuse. Preventing the disease is a different issue). Prevention programs can be found in schools, church groups, community self-help groups (not Twelve Step groups), and community clinics.

Psychiatric care may be private counseling or admission to a psychiatric unit. Dual diagnosis units are ineffective. Chemical dependency and psychiatric disorders cannot be treated simultaneously. Psychiatric wards use mind-affecting chemicals in treatment to control behavior and traditionally do not hire ex-patients to work with clients. In addition, cognitive/behavioral approaches are employed in psychiatric therapy. Chemical dependency treatment programs feature abstinence from all drugs, they hire recovered patients to aid in role-modeling and identification, and tend to stress education and personal responsibility as therapy methods. This is not to imply that some patients will not have both the disease of addiction and psychiatric problems. Some will. In this case, the primary disease determines initial treatment. If there is a question, the drug treatment center should initiate treatment, because many so-called "mental" symptoms disappear with sobriety.

On a "shotgun" unit that takes any adolescent with any drug-related problems, patients who are not really addicts will sense that they do not belong. They will placate or ignore therapists, learn the game, make fun of everything, and sabotage treatment for those who need the program.

Teenagers who really need the addiction program will get negative input from those who do not belong. Amy F., age seventeen from Littleton, Colorado shares:

> In treatment, it was hard to deal with my addiction with other adolescents who were not addicts. I would talk about how I tripped opium four times in two hours and somebody who had never even smoked pot would say, "Me too!" I needed someone to talk to about my problems, not kids who wanted to fit in and be as "bad" as I was.

Camille, age sixteen from Denver, shared her story about treatment which took place seventeen months earlier.

It was a common ritual in our treatment center—we'd tell each other our story and about our last drunk. One girl came in and we performed this ritual with her. She said, "I've only been drunk three times in my life. The reason I'm here is because I made a bet with some older guys that I'd have sex with them." She wanted recovery but she didn't belong in an alcoholic treatment center. I felt she belonged in a nut ward.

We must differentiate among adolescents who are put in treatment because their parents panicked after finding some drug paraphernalia, those ordered into treatment by the courts for delinquency, those self-medicating to control a mental problem, and those who are suffering from addiction. Accurate diagnosis is vital to successful treatment. The 1960's methods of determining drug addiction have long been outdated. Sixties parents and schools of the sixties were told to look for things like falling grades, sloppy dress, swearing, and mood swings. Since then we have learned that these are not really indicative of anything except adolescent developmental behavior. To help illustrate this see the Adolescent Drug Misuse Assessment Chart (Figure 4) on pages 62-63.

The assessment cannot be completed while teenagers are in detox under the influence of mind-affecting chemicals. At this point, testing and questionnaires are pointless and are likely to elicit nothing but disruptive and inaccurate answers. Diagnosing addiction is difficult, but it is no longer just a guessing game. Certified hospital units should take advantage of scientific methods currently available.

Researchers in Philadelphia (Mind/Addiction with George Page on educational TV, see page 71) have found a tool that can be used as a biological marker to predict alcoholism. A deficit in P-3 brain waves in response to certain stimuli has been detected in practicing alcoholics, sober alcoholics and some children of alcoholics. EEG technicians should learn to administer the test and any physician in the field of alcoholism could learn to interpret the test.

In addition, there is now a promising new blood test. This study shows that two enzymes found in blood platelet membranes react differently in alcoholics than in non-alcoholics. This test may help identify people at risk of becoming alcoholics in the early stages of drinking problems. Both of these tests have a 73 to 75 percent accuracy rate.

Hospital units charge a large sum of money to treat adolescents. There is no reason why these newest breakthroughs cannot be employed to increase their diagnostic accuracy. These types of tests added to existing diagnostic tools will make diagnosis more precise, hence increase patients' chances of recovery. Such precision may help treatment programs justify costs to insurance companies, which are increasing their scrutiny of chemical dependency programs.

Figure 4.   **ADOLESCENT DRUG MISUS**

> **NOTE**
> All of these behaviors and/or symptoms overlap into other
> areas. No category is mutually exclusive of the others.

Addiction
Blackouts
Severe Agitation
Withdrawal and Tremors
Needle Tracks
P-3 Brain Wave Deficits
Life Revolves Around Drugs
Faulty Memory
Liver Damage or Gastritis
Flagrant Disregard for Rules
Legal Problems
Violent Outbursts
Powerless To Stop Once
  Drug Is Ingested
Promiscuity

Psychological Problems
Frequent Social Isolation
Severe Mood Swings
Periods of Lethargy
Suicide Attempts or Threats
Violent Outbursts
"Crazy" Talk
Obsessed With Pornography,
  War, Paraphernalia, or
  Satanic Symbols
Anorexic or Bulimic
Severe Depressions
Bad Hygiene
Physically Harms Self

Inadequate Social Ski
Few Friends
Isolates Frequently
Not Involved In School
  Activities
May Exhibit Eating Proble
Wears Heavy Clothing To
  Hide In
Walks Hunched Over
Periods of Lethargy
Unkempt Appearance
Unable To Say No
Difficulty Accepting
  Compliments
Painfully Shy

Medical Intervention
Possible Hospitalization
Education on Disease
Therapy To Accept Disease
Funnel To AA, NA
Palmer Drug Abuse Program
School Drug-Free Support

Psychiatric Intervention
Possible Hospitalization
Therapy Groups
Follow Professional Advice

Intervention by School or
  Church
Join Youth Groups
Self Confidence Courses
Counseling at School Le
Part Time Job

> **WARNING**
> These are medical problems and
> require immediate medical attention.

> **CONSIDER**
> Any adolescent in these groups may also
> have a predisposition to the disease of
> addiction. Consider drug education
> concurrent with the above interventions.

ASSESSMENT CHART

HOW TO USE THIIS CHART

is chart will help professionals determine where to appropriately refer teenagers who have been ntified as drug users. In addition to the treatment for chemical dependents (addicts), it suggests ernative treatment modalities for those teens who misuse or abuse drugs and may have other oblems. First identify what the problem is, based upon the patient's symptoms, then determine the st course of action using your experitse and the suggestions below.

Dysfunctional Family	Drug Abuse	Normal Development
ood Swings	Sever Agitation	Mood Swings
oor Self-Image	Change in Sleeping Habits	Music Obsessions
aretaker With Friends and	Change in Friends	"Hates" Parents
Siblings	Change in Appearance	Peer Follower
arents Known Alcoholics	Drop in School Performance	Isolates in Room
equent Bruises	Preoccupation With Drugs	Prefers Friends To Family
ossible Incest	Mood Swings	Dresses Like Alien
verachiever/Underachiever	Legal Problems	Talks Like Alien
ar of Abandonment by Peers	Resentment Toward Authority	Frustrated And Petulant
annot Express Feelings	Promiscuity	Feels Picked On
gal Problems/Delinquency	Steals	Irrational
omiscuity		Won't Communicate
tremely Mature		Makes You Crazy
erfectionist		

gal or School Intervention
ssible Safe Home Placement
unseling
COA Support Group
mily Therapy

Possible Out-Patient Treatment
Counseling
Refer To Palmer Drug Abuse
  Program
Education on Disease

CAUTION
Sometimes it is difficult to distinguish between temporary development stages of drug abuse and the initital stages of drug addiction. Therefore you may want to closely observe this adolescent as a candidate for ten day in-patient chemical dependency evaluation.

PARENTAL RESPONSE
Remain Firm
Set Limits
Do Not Accept Abuse
Wait Until They're Thirty

Rules and Regulations

Imagine you are sick, coming off drugs. You have gotten into trouble and landed in treatment behind locked doors. The hospital staff says, "No smoking, no cookies, candy, potato chips, no coffee, tea, or Pepsi, no contact with the opposite sex." Then they inform you that you are going to learn how to live a sober, happy life.

Would you believe them? Adolescents do not believe them, either. With a program like this, you lose before you begin. Many programs are run just this restrictively. Such an approach is not accidental; there are logical reasons why these rules developed.

Before the Eighties, there were very few treatment centers that addressed adolescents specifically. Adult treatment was just coming out of the dark ages, when alcoholics were refused admittance to hospitals and shock treatments were administered as "cures." Practitioners were just learning, among other things, that to have any type of recovery success, they must funnel their patients into continuing support groups like Alcoholics Anonymous and Narcotics Anonymous.

Then the medical profession noticed that people under the age of twenty-five could be just as sick with alcoholism/addiction as adults. Demand for treatment from terrified parents and court systems trying to break criminal patterns in youth necessitated treatment for young adults and adolescents. There were no model programs—no bad programs to avoid, no good programs to emulate.

There was no place specifically for teens except adolescent psychiatric wards. Unfortunately, most of the current treatment centers for teens were modeled after these wards. Even the staff was recruited from these programs because few professionals from other disciplines had experience with adolescents. It seemed an easy solution. Take the staff from adolescent psych wards, combine that with drug education, behavioral techniques, and adapt both to meet insurance requirements. However hopeful it may have appeared at the time, it did not work.

The disease of addiction is not a mental disorder or behavior problem, and most psychiatric wards are designed to treat mental disorders behaviorally. With their levels, phases, demerits, and behavior modification techniques, professionals seem to be saying that teaching teens to behave in an "hospital appropriate" manner will help their addiction "get better."

One program I visited in Texas handed out thirty-eight typed pages of instructions, rules, policies, and expectations for the adolescent. It included:

> Dress code: girls have to wear bras, no cut offs, no Rock T-shirts, no tight clothes, no hats, no dangling earrings;

> Contraband: candy, gum, belts with buckles, keys, driver's license, bank books, posters;

> Limited: all phone calls to five minutes, visits by family, no contact with the opposite sex.

Also included in the instructions were five pages of unit policies and rules with the apology: "We have attempted to minimize the number of policies as much as possible." This seems so far from the truth that the inconsistency alone would force a patient to "tune out" anything else the program had to say. This is not unlike a teen who gets misinformation about drugs from a parent or school and no longer listens to the information that is correct.

Jeanette, a teenager from Thousand Oaks, California, says:

> My father is a policeman. He told me and my brothers that "one shot of heroin and you're hooked for life." I loved, respected and believed him. But then I met people who chippied with heroin for years. I knew my father had lied or was terribly misinformed himself. So I stopped listening to anything he had to say about drugs from then on.

This same thirty-eight page document also had a section on the patient's responsibilities which asked a patient who felt violated to inform the staff in writing. Since many teens feel inadequate about their writing skills or can be illiterate, this is unrealistic.

Another treatment center I worked with in Denver had a similar thirty-five page document. Almost every adolescent unit is the same around the country. We cannot regulate and control a child's natural growth patterns. For example, teenagers are developing sexually and rules about not speaking to or contacting the opposite sex are unrealistic.

Pubertal processes cannot be controlled. It is important to teenage recovery to address these issues, not deny them.

At this time in their lives, teens are developing individuality, finding out how they are different, and exploring the beauty of their uniqueness. Simultaneously, they want to be loved and accepted; they want to explore being different. The following chart contrasts natural maturation with inappropriate treatment procedures:

DEVELOPMENT	NEED TO	Rx SUPPRESSES
Sexuality	Accept male/female-ness, explore intimacy, love and be loved	No touching, talking to the opposite sex, or dating
Independence	Start being responsible, accept consequences	Parents pay for Rx, constant controls, ACOA and CoDA overdone
Individuality	Find own style	With dress codes, with music codes, verbal restrictions
Testing Adult World	Drink coffee, talk with adults, test adult habits	No coffee or sugar, segregation, no smoking

This is by no means all-inclusive. You can probably add many more examples from your own observations.

The teen is not a child anymore. The disease has propelled him or her into a more serious position. Neither is he or she an adult. Teen addicts are facing life and death issues and are forced to make life and death decisions. We cannot protect them from that situation. We have to convince them of it. Mike C., age sixteen from Littleton, Colorado, says:

> It doesn't matter if you swear, listen to heavy metal, wear ratty clothes, or have long hair. If you want to quit you will. Your appearance has nothing to do with your recovery. They tried to tell me in treatment this was important but I knew it wasn't. Going to meetings, staying away from drugs, having fun—that's what's important.

In the book *Tough Love,* the Palmer Drug Abuse Program is said to use a hospital that has three basic rules:

No coming to meetings high or using.

No sex or sexual acting-out.

No violence.

It makes sense. As professionals, we cannot give teens back their childhood and we are not their parents. We do not need to baby-sit, discipline, smother, make excuses, or mete out punishment. We have to help heal and impart knowledge and understanding, not control behavior, make rules, or pass judgments.

Mainstreaming

In the history of adolescent drug treatment, the first unfortunate program strategy was to glean techniques and staff from psychiatric units. The second unfortunate decision was to segregate and isolate young people in recovery.

Mac McFadden, founder and director of The Ark in Green Mountain, Colorado, has some interesting things to say regarding segregation of patients:

> We are treating an illness here. We're not treating adolescents, blacks, women—those entities are not diseases. If they were, we would treat them. We are treating an illness and it doesn't change from one group to the next.

From personal observation, most of the recovering adolescents who have remained sober after treatment went through adult units. I am not totally discounting adolescent units, but there are several good reasons to reevaluate their overall effectiveness.

On an adolescent ward, staff often have unconscious prejudices (see Chapter 4, Habit or Disease). People feel that teens "Can't possibly be that sick yet," or "They're potential addicts." These subtle messages are conveyed to young patients and their parents, thus no one takes the disease as seriously as they should. On an adult unit, no one questions (even subconsciously) the seriousness of the disease. The message going to adult patients gets through to the adolescents and they begin their recovery with the same seriousness as the adults around them.

In an adult center, teens learn to communicate their feelings to adults. Mac McFadden explains:

> Teenagers have trouble communicating feelings to their parents—something they desperately need to learn for recovery. In a multi-aged treatment milieu, the teen has an older roommate whom he "communicates" with. Since they're both struggling in treatment with heavy issues, they share feelings. Then they go to group and since the teen has opened up with one adult, he opens up in group. At the same time, as treatment provider, we communicate with their parents. Then we get the teen and parent together and since the kid has opened up with adults in group, he or she feels more capable of communicating with parents. That chance is not available in peer treatment.

On adolescent units, the focus is diverted from treatment. Debra Gray Hogan, CD counselor from Abaris in Beloit, Wisconsin explains:

> I like adolescents treated with adults because I don't like what happens when units fill up with mostly kids. All of a sudden we're dealing with behavior problems and worrying about them making their beds. We worry about their music and clothes. We become baby-sitters. They're making out in the lounge and we're saying "Don't do this and don't do that." The caretaking becomes the focus instead of treatment of the disease.

On adolescent units, negative bonding occurs. Teens tend to reinforce their own bad habits. They use slang that excludes the staff, make fun of the programs and staff, and constantly try to impress each other at the center's expense. They group together and decide they know better than the staff. Shannon Goatz, CTRS at Porter's Centre in Denver, says:

> Teens get into negative bonding and start the "us against them" syndrome. When teenagers are mainstreamed with adults, we don't have these negative bonding problems. For instance, in adult treatment there is no such thing as a "runaway." There are patients who leave treatment against medical advice but this is not a regular occurrence because adults don't see it as "cool" to run off.

On adolescent units, everything becomes an "issue." There is the clothing issue, phone calls, romances, music, posters, punk hair styles, runaways... and in response to all this, levels, phases and reward systems are enacted to control the "issues."

The best reason to re-evaluate the effectiveness of segregation is that my recent experience shows that mainstreaming works better for adolescents. Psychologist Dr. Michael Marshall and I surveyed 100 clean and sober people who had gone for treatment as adolescents. The study "Homogeneous Versus Heterogeneous Age Group Treatment of Adolescent Substance Abusers" (which simply means: teens treated with teens-only versus teens treated with adults) soon to be published in *The American Journal Of Alcohol And Drug Abuse*, suggests that adolescents treated with adults are four to five times more likely to recover than those treated in adolescent-only centers (see Appendix 3).

The peer pressure in adult centers is "mature" in nature contrasted to the pressure on an adolescent-only unit. If a problem does occur, say a girl is dressing too suggestively for other patients' comfort, it is handled on a one-to-one basis. This is how it would be handled with any adult who does something that makes others uncomfortable.

Kevin O. from Denver, twenty-two years old with four years sobriety, says:

> It was encouraging to see other teenage alcoholics sober but it was also encouraging to meet and get to know older recovered alcoholics because it made me feel as though I was growing. I was glad I was able to interact with all ages in treatment because somehow it made me feel more responsible for my recovery.

Chad E. from Lakewood, Colorado speaks of the main argument against mainstreaming teens:

> I did an internship at a treatment center where they split the unit into adult and adolescent units. The reason given for this was that it prevented the adults from manipulating and taking advantage of the young people. But with proper supervision, I do believe that adults and adolescents can mix effectively.

Professionals and other staff should be aware of manipulative behavior such as conning the younger patients out of money, favors, and making sexual advances. But remember, we are not dealing with the world's innocents here. It is also likely that some teens will manipulate adults.

Linda Yoakem suggests:

Perhaps have separate sleeping quarters, but identical day-time treatment. The biggest argument I have heard against mainstreamed treatment is parents' fears that their child will be sexually violated by an adult. Insurance and legal issues get into this as well. If a sexual incident occurs between an adolescent and an adult while under the supervision of a treatment center, lawsuits can happen. Treatment centers are terrified of this.

And justifiably so. But more disturbing is treatment that does not work when people's lives are at stake. Mainstreaming adolescents is also less expensive than adolescent-only units. The staff/patient ratio has to be higher in adolescent units to control behavior and the stays are longer (adults generally stay twenty-eight days to the adolescents' forty-five days). Basically we as professionals cannot afford to ignore this question of mainstreaming any longer. Adolescents are not recovering in the same numbers as adults. Treat them with adults and they will recover at the same rate as everyone else.

Chapter Highlights

1. In the assessment period of detox, we must weed out those that do not have the disease of addiction. Treating drug-abusing teens with behavior problems is not treatment, it is prevention. Treatment for psychiatric disorders should be separate from chemical dependency treatment. Both require different approaches than that used in treatment of the incurable and chronic disease of addiction.

2. Too many rules and regulations divert the program focus from what should be going on in treatment. Treatment centers should focus on treatment, not caretaking.

3. Adult treatment centers impress adolescents with the truth: they have an adult disease. This enables them to take their recovery as seriously as any adult.

4. Research suggests that mainstreaming adolescents with adults gives them their best chance at recovery.

Resources

Books

Dolan, J. *I Never Saw The Sun Rise*. Minneapolis: Comp Care Publishers, 1977.

Baron, J.D. *The Parents' Handbook of Drug Abuse and Treatment*, Houston: DAPA, 1981.

Research

Nehr, T. 1991. Altered States. *Professional Counselor* 5: 31-35.

Tabakoff, B. et al. 1988. Alcoholism; A New and Promising Blood Test. *New England Journal of Medicine*. 318: 134.

Videos

George Page, *Mind/Addiction* (volume 4), WNET/New York: Educational Broadcasting Corporation, 1988.

Chapter 6

The Content of Treatment

Most chemically dependent teenagers do not enter treatment because they want to stop using chemicals. They come to treatment because they want bad things to stop happening to them. They want parents and school off their backs. They do not want to go to jail, lose their driver's license, or have friends reject them. Hence one of the first and most important steps in in-patient treatment is to help teenagers realize that they really need treatment. They need to know they have an illness that is ruining their lives. Often, realizing this goal takes up most of the treatment process.

We know that chemical dependency is a primary disease. It is not a symptom of a deeper underlying problem; it is the problem. It causes a myriad of other symptoms like emotional troubles, physical illness, poor family relations, and abusive personalities. None of these issues can be addressed until the primary disease is treated.

As long as we professionals remember this, we will not be tempted to sidetrack what needs to be addressed in the treatment of the teenager. Although most issues to be addressed are no different from those of adults, certain areas should be differentiated while the teen is mainstreamed. This is called teen tracking. We will examine practical examples of teen tracking that can be used in treatment centers.

Three areas are critical with in-patient and out-patient treatment: habilitation, education and acceptance of the disease, and parents and other enablers. There are only slight differences between treatment of teens and adults in these areas.

Habilitation

Teens are not *rehabilitated* in the same way as adults. Teenagers are *habilitated.* They have not had time to mature before being interrupted by the disease. Therefore, what adults are relearning, adolescents are learning for the first time.

Emotional development is halted or stunted at the onset of drug use. This means that if teens began using at age ten or eleven and they recover at age fourteen or fifteen, they will still have to go through puberty. Part of recovery is helping them through that process.

Many adult alcoholics remember the "Good Old Days" before they used or when drinking and marijuana still worked for them. Teens do not have those memories. They probably never learned adequate social skills and still have this learning process ahead of them. This can actually work to the benefit of treatment staff. If you are mainstreaming your adolescents, you will have the experience of the adult patients to aid you. Teach the adults how to practice their previous living skills as you teach the teens these skills for the first time. These include: communication skills with family, friends, and authority figures, assertiveness techniques, and whatever else your center chooses to emphasize in treatment.

A patient's life cannot be reorganized in thirty to forty-five days, so the treatment program should include an aftercare program. Part of aftercare includes funnelling adolescents into AA, NA, CA, and PDAP. Research shows that in order for the rate of recovery to improve, patients must be socialized into a Twelve Step program of recovery—*it is the single most important part of your treatment.* All treatment can do is get people started in the recovery process by getting the drugs out of them long enough so they may make a decision to save their lives. Camille, age sixteen from Denver, says:

> Treatment gave me forty-five days of sobriety and clean time. I don't think I could have achieved those first few weeks without it. It

also introduced me to a Twelve Step program without which I wouldn't have had any sobriety or clean time at all.

Although the desire of professionals is to have greater control and direct influence on their patients' recovery process, this hope is unrealistic. The four significant things they may achieve be:

Convincing teenagers they have the disease of addiction.

Educating teens about the disease.

Showing teenagers what the disease has done and will do to them.

Getting teenagers to accept a Twelve Step program for a lifetime of sobriety.

This is what treatment did for Melonie H., from Colorado Springs, sober two years:

> I had a real hard time believing that I was an alcoholic when I first came around because I was nineteen years old. Most of the people I saw were quite a bit older than me. I have never had a DUI or been in prison, I've never lost a home or a family, but for me I had to realize that those were all of my "yets." If I continued to drink, all of those things would happen to me. I think other teens do not get sober because they do not take sobriety seriously. They think none of those things will happen to them.

If we can persuade teenagers to accept their disease and its seriousness and get them dedicated to a Twelve Step program, habilitation has begun. This still leaves two areas of habilitation that any treatment center with people under the age of twenty should address: peer pressure and parties; sex and dating in the recovery process.

Peer Pressure and Parties

Peer pressure is an ugly issue because teenagers react violently when they are told the truth:

You cannot hang out with your old friends who use drugs, drink alcohol, or smoke marijuana—not for one day, one party, one hour. You will not stay clean and sober if you suffer from the delusion that you can safely do this.

Practitioners and parents have a hard time conveying this message because teens simply do not want to believe it. They think they are stronger than they actually are. Adolescents often want to stay sober, but falsely believe they can watch their friends drink while they themselves turn down alcohol. Professionals know better and have to convince young clients of the truth. Adolescents feel they are being disloyal to drop friends after treatment, but the job is to convince them true loyalty lies with themselves and a Higher Power.

On the peer pressure and party issues, be strong; play dirty; tell horror stories; get speakers to tell about their problems with "using" friends. Get clients to read the real life stories of recovering youth from *Young, Sober, & Free*. Do not let any adolescent leave your center with even a glimmer of hope that he or she can keep drug-using friends, because they cannot. It does not work. It is not professionally responsible to allow young patients or their parents to think that it will.

Sex and dating

It is the task of every teen to learn to belong and to accept their sexuality. Dealing with polarity (male/female) is an enormous task on the way to adulthood. Teens need to explore and experience intimacy and develop the capacity to love and be loved by others.

Never tell young adults they cannot date, have sex, or masturbate in order to stay sober. It is not true and will only instill guilt about things they are going to do anyway. Such admonitions jeopardize their recovery. Chris Hartlep, a chemical dependency counselor from Beloit, Wisconsin talks about moralizing on sexual issues:

> On sexual and other standards: what's normal in Beloit may not be normal in California. A real struggle I had was learning about abnormal behavior. There's a lot of literature on that. But where's the section on what's normal? And what's culturally normal concerning sex? I don't know.

Be open and honest about personal beliefs but make it clear that those beliefs are your own. All addicts will have to come to terms with their own sexuality. The facts about AIDS, contraception, the sex act, and orgasm should be taught. We must erase guilt over past degrading sexual behavior and help them reject it as a way of life. Expecting a streetwise, drug wise addict to revert to cartoons on Saturday night and suddenly pretend she is a virgin will not work.

Education And Acceptance
Of The Disease

One of the easiest methods of getting patients to accept their disease is to surround them with peers who already accept it. This is most readily accomplished by socialization into the Twelve Step groups of recovery. The best idea I have encountered for beginning this process comes from Spring Shadows Glen, Houston, Texas. Patient committees are organized and governed in the same manner as a Twelve Step group. Gwen Hettinger, program coordinator explains:

The principles of the Twelve Steps of AA, and many other self-help groups, are one of the basic concepts of our treatment program. Throughout a patient's stay, we continually stress the long-term benefits of using the AA philosophy in all the affairs of life.

One method of doing this is by organizing the patient's self-government committee along the lines of an AA type group. As you know, there are no "presidents" etc., but rather chairpersons and leaders to guide and facilitate regular meetings. Many groups also have additional offices to handle finance and other necessary duties so that the group can regularly meet for the sole purpose of maintaining sobriety.

The patient committee functions only in the areas of community meetings, patient meetings or special functions. All of their decisions/actions are within hospital rules and guidelines. They may, however, petition the staff on specific matters.

Figure 5 lists the patient committee positions, duties, and requirements.

Adolescents leaving this hospital are not confused about the structure of AA and are trained to participate in the appropriate organization for them. Patient committees patterned after AA steering committees give a tremendous advantage to anyone, especially youth not accustomed to self-government.

Figure 5.

Patient Committee

Members: Chairperson, Leader, Secretary, Treasurer, Steering Committee (two), Special Events Chairperson, Patient Greeters (two)

CHAIRPERSON (chosen)

Qualifications: Working on or completed Step Three, working avidly with a sponsor, good attitude, walking not talking, and preparing for discharge. Chairperson to be appointed by Medical Director, Program Coordinator, and Nursing Coordinator on recommendation by all staff.

Duties: Opens community meeting (AA fashion), chairs and leads Friday night business meeting, assists new officers, and orients new officers, examines and introduces all unit proposals, liaises with counselors for Twelve Step meetings on campus and leads the community meeting in the absence of the meeting leader.

LEADER (elected)

Qualifications: Working on or completed Step Two, knowledge of Robert's Rules of Order, working with a sponsor, minimum of three weeks of off-grounds meetings, a positive attitude.

Duties: Responsible for maintaining and leading community meetings, liaison to unit staff and chairs meeting in chairperson's absence.

SECRETARY (elected)

Qualifications: Completed Step One, working in all areas of treatment.

Duties: Takes minutes of all meetings, responsible for secretary reports. Responsible for having current list of proposals for nursing.

TREASURER (elected)

Qualifications: Completed Step One, working in all areas of treatment.

Duties: Responsible for events involving funding and coordinating these with staff. Keeps pantry food list. Fills in for secretaries in their absence.

STEERING COMMITTEE (two) (elected)

Qualifications: Completed Step One, minimum of one week off-grounds meetings, and positive attitude.

Duties: Set-up for all patient activities, in charge of clean up and line up.

SPECIAL EVENTS CHAIRPERSON (elected)

Qualifications: Completed Step One, working in all areas of treatment.

Duties: Coordinating any and all special events with leader, treasurer, and staff.

PATIENT GREETERS (elected) as per patient greeter guide.

"We are but trusted servants, and our common welfare must come first."

Another way to encourage teens to accept their disease requires more subtlety. It is called "dealing with the informal psyche." Young adults like to exhibit what they believe in and make statements to the world about who they are. Thus, they display drug culture T-shirts, jewelry, belt buckles, hats. Replace these with sobriety symbols. Have sober T-shirts, jewelry, cups, hats, etc., and make them available to the kids. Have them design their own. But remember—messages should be humorous, "awesome," or "bad", not moralizing, religious, preachy, or hokey.

Education about the disease is one of the most important aspects of treatment. For the adolescent, there can be several barriers to this process. These can include vocabulary problems, learning disabilities, or borderline illiteracy. Few of us realize that our patients may not even understand what we are talking about.

Have fun with them. Be creative. Take chances. If what you have done in the past is not working, try new and innovative approaches. Terri Wilkes, a youth recovery facilitator from Georgia shares her ideas:

> During my eight years of working with teenagers in Twelve Step recovery programs, I found more and more a lack of interest in learning the Twelve Steps of AA. I tried several approaches to get the teenagers to learn what was, I felt, a road map to their new life. I tried study groups, study time alone and pairing the teenagers in teams to help each other. Each time ended the same—those motivated to recover studied and learned, but the less interested played. I decided there must be a "fun" way of learning. I got the idea of the Twelve Step Jumble (Figure 6) and used it as a group activity allowing the teenagers to use the Big Book. After everyone had completed the Jumble, the group took turns in reading the unscrambled step and the number. As I facilitated, I saw participation and interest, and it was "fun." It worked.

Finally, some of the words teens are frequently not familiar with include but are not limited to: powerless, stereotype, intimacy, masculinity, femininity, principles, tolerance, occupational, syndrome, blackout, anxiety, anonymous, meditation, etc.

Kay Nightingale, a certified teacher, education specialist, and the school system's Substance Abuse Coordinator in Beloit, Wisconsin, is developing a unique concept for adolescents in treatment. She has designed several curriculum methods to be used in the required schooling for teens in treatment based on the text and stories of *Young, Sober, &*

Free. This way, young addicts will be earning required credits while learning about their disease. This is what Ms. Nightingale has to say:

> The educational program is most meaningful when integrated into the total treatment program. Reading about the disease, developing vocabulary and literature around the disease concept and recovery stories will offer an integrated approach to the educational component of treatment. Emphasis needs to be on initiating or fostering a positive attitude about the adolescent's academic ability and capability, with attention paid to the importance of completing his or her education as an integral part of recovery. Saying "yes" to education will help the recovering adolescent say "no" to using.

The value of combining schooling with alcoholism/addiction education helps reinforce the whole treatment milieu for teens. The educational literature written for adults can be revised to incorporate adolescents' language and teen circumstances. Instead of "spouse," use "parents" and "siblings"; instead of a "job," refer to "school"; instead of "cocktail parties," use "keggers". (See Figure 7, the recovery graph for adults and compare it to the same graph modified for use by adolescents, Figure 8.)

Figure 6.

Twelve Step Jumble

1. ____ made over will care a decision and lives to the turn our to and of him understand God as we

2. ____ character all of these God defects remove entirely to have ready were

3. ____ others made or direct amends them injure to such would people so do to wherever when except possible

4. ____ we unmanageable become alcohol admitted had lives over powerless our were we that

5. ____ power greater came to that believe a sanity than ourselves could restore us to

6. ____ made ourselves a fearless of a inventory moral and searching

7. ____ sought out that carry through prayer and to meditation power to the improve and us for our will conscious his contact with of God knowledge for only as we praying understood him

8. ____ wrongs admitted our of to God nature to ourselves exact and the to being another human

9. ____ humbly shortcoming our asked him to remove

10.____ continued wrong personal promptly to take we were inventory admitted it and when

11.____ spiritual awakening having had in all our affairs as the principles result these of these steps we tried practice to and to carry   alcoholics to message this a

12.____ made a to them all list of all amends persons make we had harmed and to willing became

Instructions: Unscramble the words to complete the steps. Fill in the blank to the correct number of that step.

Figure 7.

Addiction And Recovery

HEAVY USE BEGINS

OCCASIONAL RELIEF DRINKING

INCREASING TOLERANCE

BEHAVIOR CHANGES

MEMORY BLACKOUTS

RELATIONSHIPS SUFFER

DECREASE OF ATTENTION SPAN AND LOW FRUSTRATION LEVEL

REMORSE

BLAMES OTHERS FOR OWN TROUBLES

PROMISES AND RESOLUTIONS FAIL

MONDAY AND FRIDAY ABSENTEEISM AT WORK

DWI'S & LEGAL PROBLEMS

TRIES GEOGRAPHICAL CURES

PREOCCUPATION WITH DRUG OF CHOICE

FAMILY AND FRIENDS AVOIDED IF NOT USING DRUGS

PERSONAL HYGIENE DETERIORATES

UNREASONABLE RESENTMENT

WORK AND MONEY TROUBLES

NEGLECT OF FOOD

ONSET OF LENGTHY INTOXICATION

PHYSICAL DETERIORATION

UNPREDICTABLE OUTCOME TO USE

DRINKING OR USING WITH INFERIORS

IMPAIRED THINKING

UNABLE TO INITIATE ACTION

ALL ALIBIS EXHAUSTED

INDEFINABLE FEARS

OBSESSION WITH USE

VAGUE DESIRE FOR HELP

COMPLETE DEFEAT ADMITTED

HONEST DESIRE FOR HELP

TOLD ADDICTION CAN BE ARRESTED

MEETS NORMAL AND HAPPY FORMER ADDICTS

STOPS TAKING MIND ALTERING CHEMICALS

ASSISTED IN HONEST SELF APPRAISAL

PHYSICAL EXAMINATION BY DOCTOR

RIGHT THINKING BEGINS

START OF GROUP THERAPY

SPIRITUAL NEEDS EXAMINED

ONSET OF NEW HOPE

REGULAR NOURISHMENT TAKEN

NORMAL GROOMING RETURNS

WELCOMES RECOVERY

RETURN OF SELF-ESTEEM

REALISTIC THINKING

NATURAL REST AND SLEEP

FAMILY AND FRIENDS APPRECIATE EFFORT

ADJUSTMENT TO FAMILY NEEDS

NEW CIRCLE OF FRIENDS

NEW INTERESTS DEVELOP

INCREASE OF EMOTIONAL CONTROL

REBIRTH OF INTEGRITY

STEPS TOWARD ECONOMIC STABILITY

CONFIDENCE OF EMPLOYER

BEGINS TO REACH OUT TO OTHERS IN 12TH STEP WORK

TRUST OF FRIENDS REGAINED

ASSUMES FULL RESPONSIBILITY FOR TROUBLES

ENLIGHTENED AND INTERESTING LIFE OPENS UP WITH SOBRIETY

COMMITMENT TO SOBRIETY

AA & NA

Adolescent Addiction And Recovery

Addiction (descending):

HEAVY USE BEGINS

EXPERIMENTAL DRUG USE

KNOWN CHEMICAL DEPENDENCY IN FAMILY

INCREASING TOLERANCE

BEHAVIOR CHANGES

MEMORY BLACKOUTS

REBUFFS PARENTS

INATTENTIVENESS IN CLASS AND ANGERS EASILY

BLAMES OTHERS FOR OWN TROUBLES

WIDE MOOD SWINGS

MONDAY AND FRIDAY TRUANCIES AT SCHOOL

BEGINS TO LIE AND SNEAK

TRUENCY AND DETENTION

DISCONTINUES EXTRACURRICULAR ACTIVITIES

INCREASED NEED FOR IMMEDIATE HIGH

FAMILY AND FRIENDS AVOIDED IF NOT USING DRUGS

BEGINS TO LOOK AND SMELL DIRTY

UNREASONABLE RESENTMENT

MAKING SCENES IN SCHOOL

NEGLECT OF FOOD

ONSET OF LENGTHY HIGHS

BODY FALLS APART

UNPREDICTABLE OUTCOME TO USE

ASSOCIATES WITH DRUG SUBCULTURE

SCREWY THINKING

NO INTEREST IN SCHOOL OR FAMILY ACTIVITIES

INDEFINABLE FEARS

ALL EXCUSES GONE

OBSESSION WITH USE

VAGUE DESIRE FOR HELP

COMPLETE DEFEAT ADMITTED

HITS BOTTOM

Recovery (ascending):

HONEST DESIRE FOR HELP

TOLD THERE IS AN ANSWER

MEETS NORMAL AND HAPPY FORMER ADDICTS

STOPS TAKING MIND ALTERING CHEMICALS

PHYSICAL EXAMINATION BY DOCTOR

ASSISTED IN HONEST SELF APPRAISAL

HEAD STRAIGHTENS OUT

START OF GROUP THERAPY

SPIRITUAL NEEDS EXAMINED

ONSET OF NEW HOPE

EATING REGULAR AGAIN

NORMAL GROOMING RETURNS

WELCOMES RECOVERY

BEGINS TO REALLY LIKE SELF

REALISTIC THINKING

NATURAL REST AND SLEEP

FAMILY APPRECIATES EFFORT

NEW CIRCLE OF FRIENDS

ADJUSTMENT TO FAMILY NEEDS

INCREASE OF EMOTIONAL CONTROL

NEW INTERESTS DEVELOP

RESUMES INTEREST IN FUTURE

BEGINS TO TRUST SELF

BEGINS TO REACH OUT TO OTHERS IN 12TH STEP WORK

RETURN TO SCHOOL OR JOB

ASSUMES FULL RESPONSIBILITY FOR TROUBLES

TRUST OF FRIENDS REGAINED

ENLIGHTENED AND INTERESTING LIFE OPENS UP WITH SOBRIETY

COMMITMENT TO SOBRIETY

AA & NA

Parents And Other Enablers

The involvement of the entire family is not essential but is desirable. The disease of one family member has a definite impact on the entire family and involvement by the family has a significant effect on the recovery process. However, it is important to let the adolescent know that regardless of his family's chosen involvement—he or she can recover.

Unfortunately, teens have many more enablers than do adult alcoholic/addicts. The enablers are parents, teachers, uncles, grandparents, the local police officer who is everyone's buddy, well-meaning friends of troubled parents, and the parents of friends. Ultimately, the adolescent will have to recognize the pitfalls of the well-intended enablers in his or her life. The younger a person is when he or she begins recovery, the greater the obstacles they will encounter in society. As the addicts grow older, people who have never seen them use drugs will not believe they have a disease. People who have seen them use drugs will think they were "too young" to have really been sick. Suddenly, the recovering young people are pressured by countless people in their lives to "just have one," or "stop pretending to be an addict," or "stop trying to get attention by using drugs." My own history of sobriety from age twenty-one illustrates this:

> The first few years everyone who had known me was terribly grateful I was sober and not dead. But at around five years of sobriety people started expressing disbelief that I was really an addict/alcoholic. Boyfriends tried to get me to drink and smoke pot. After ten years, my old friends forgot how sick I had been and "humored" me about my alcoholism, Twelve Step meetings, and Twelve Step work. It was terribly frustrating. At nineteen years sobriety my new husband and my daughter did not believe I was an alcoholic. Of course they had no comparison from the past because they had always known me sober. It just showed their ignorance about alcoholism, but if my program or conscious contact had been weak, I might have been tempted to listen to them. I have talked to other people who acquired sobriety young and have over fifteen years success. The story is the same—so many of us are told that we "couldn't possibly be" by well-meaning people or that we are making our history of addiction up because it's the "in" thing today.

"Burn the idea into the consciousness of every man that he can get well regardless of anyone" (*Alcoholics Anonymous*, page 98). Burn the idea into the consciousness of every teenager that he or she can get well regardless of anyone or anything—best friend, peers, boyfriends and girlfriends, brothers and sisters, Dad's drinking, Mom's abusiveness, the pressures of school, and well-meaning misinformed people who say "You're too young to be an alcoholic."

Chapter Highlights

1. In treatment we can really only accomplish four things:

   Convince adolescents they have the disease.

   Show adolescents exactly what that disease is.

   Show adolescents what the disease has done and will do to them.

   Get adolescents to accept a Twelve Step program for a lifetime of sobriety.

2. Do not give a glimmer of hope to the adolescent that he or she can hang out with old drug friends. However much they fight you, you must never let them believe they can remain clean and be with their old friends for one day, one party or one hour. We know it does not work.

3. Burn the idea into the mind of every recovering teen that he or she can stay clean regardless of the situation at home, regardless of peers, regardless of the uninformed people who will try to convince them they are too young to be an alcoholic/addict.

Resources

Books

Alcoholics Anonymous. NY: AA World Services, Inc., 1939.

Narcotics Anonymous. Van Nuys: NA World Services, Inc., 1982.

Marshall, Shelly. *Young, Sober, & Free.* Center City, Minnesota: Hazelden Publishing, 1978.

Periodicals

Kepp, Kritdine. 1988. Sexual Acting Out. *Adolescent Counselor* Oct/Nov.

Chapter 7

Skills of the Staff

It is inappropriate to speak about the skills of the staff without first speaking about the skills of the people who hire them. This includes the program directors, corporate executives, and nursing supervisors who run the program. Those in charge want to protect their jobs but they also want to find meaning in their careers.

Successful treatment centers can give directors, executives, and supervisors a sense of fulfillment. Only in the centers where adolescents maintain sobriety will the staff get that wonderful sense of meaning. The opportunity for us to excel in our field begins with the people we hire, the criteria we use to find them, and how honest we are with ourselves about what traits facilitate working with people effectively.

It is important to ferret out the professional discrepancies and hidden prejudices in the people working with us. It is important to hire professionals who believe addiction is a disease. Professionals who cannot accept that adolescents can be as seriously sick as adult patients will inhibit the adolescent's recovery. If this type of professional already works for you, try to set up in-house training or staff therapy sessions to deal with the problem.

Let me share an experience my daughter and I had:

> After my daughter had been in treatment for three weeks, I found out she really did not like her psychiatrist. "What's the problem?" I asked.
>
> "Oh, he keeps saying it's a joke on us. That you're the big expert on teenage alcoholism and now I'm an alcoholic and the joke's on you."

Because she is an alcoholic (they lie and manipulate), I checked with several other staff about her allegations and learned that the psychiatrist had made numerous remarks like that.

This clearly demonstrated that the psychiatrist did not understand the biological nature of the disease. I told her to ask him if it was a joke on an oncologist if his child got melanoma. She did and he stopped his remarks.

But patients, whether adolescent or otherwise, should never have to disagree with the staff about what the disease is and isn't. It is the director's responsibility to assure that the staff will never put their patients in such a position.

Also avoid hiring people with "related degrees" just because they have experience working with adolescents. Psychology majors, social workers, and psychiatric nurses are not necessarily qualified to work on a chemical dependency unit because they have a parallel degree or because they have previously worked with adolescents. The most important qualification is that they know about addiction or are willing to learn.

Imagine you have children with leukemia on a unit. You need an RN to run things. You would not hire the RN who had been a school nurse, you would hire the RN who had been an oncologist's assistant. It would be nice if the RN had expertise with children as well, but you need the expertise in cancer, not kids.

Adolescence is not the disease. Hiring professionals with parallel degrees who have worked with teens results in reward/punishment treatment for teens where the teens work up the levels through a behavior modification approach. Behavior modification does not work with addicted adults and it does not work with addicted teenagers. Make sure before hiring professionals that they know they are not treating a behavior problem.

When hiring staff, directors should also consider some seemingly superficial characteristics that may strongly influence their teen patients.

Size

Yes, actual physical size. The bigger a man or woman is, the more likely a teen is to respond to them. I do not have an explanation for this, however, it is observable. Tall or wide, the bigger, the better.

Badness

Bikers, the streetwise, ex-gang members, tough minorities, tough females...they like the flair; it seems glamorous, they respond to it.

Extremes of age

Adolescents admire other youth in positions of authority. They also respond well to the very old. You would be surprised how a seventy year old extending a loving hand can elicit positive responses from teenagers.

Humor

Brings out the best in every patient. If you get the chance to get a real clown or comedian on your unit, go for it. They sometimes do not take you seriously enough, but if you can handle their antics, they will really help improve the therapeutic atmosphere.

Pathos

Someone who can make them cry, who has had tough breaks they can share with the kids. Teenagers like underdogs and if you have a staff member that couples competence with a sympathy evoking story that person can really improve the therapeutic relationship. Hire the handicapped, ex-skid row people, minorities.

Fame

Yes, it's true. Teens like the feeling of being close to anyone who was ever someone—ex-sports personalities, rock stars, authors, any type of celebrity. You may not be so lucky as to have them apply, but they do exist and if you get an opportunity, hire them.

I am not suggesting that just because someone exhibits these characteristics, they should be hired. They also must be qualified. Work with your existing staff as well. Try not to force them into the middle class, American suit and briefcase mold. If you have staff members with more flair or you have a chance to hire someone in leather, it will not hurt your program. It may enhance it.

Finally, allowing your staff the space to be creative and innovative will let them pour their hearts into their job. Most people want to pour their hearts into it, but if corporate policy or inflexible programming stifles personnel, it stifles the whole treatment atmosphere.

Linda Yoakem, M.S. in clinical psychology, shares her experiences:

After my education was completed, I worked for a private treatment center developing an out-patient adolescent program. I had some real problems with the discrepancy between the verbal and written expectations of me and the actual duties I was expected to perform. For instance, I stressed during my employment interview that I wanted to be creative and innovative in developing the program. The interviewer agreed but when it came to the way I was expected to run things, I was pressured to stick to the program already in use.

Another problem that I encountered with the program was diagnosis according to ability to pay. I saw individuals who needed treatment desperately either turned away or put in a program which did not meet the needs of the client strictly because they did not have insurance. I also saw individuals who were from financially secure families placed in intensive treatment when there was no need for it, they were only abusing drugs, not addicted. I had a teen in my group verbalize to me that out-patient treatment was not working for him, but was discouraged by my superiors when I tried to get the individual into in-patient treatment. I was told such things as "give out-patient a chance to work" (it obviously was not working), or " there are no beds available in our in-patient program" (What about other programs? Oh, that would be losing revenue for our program). So the teen was kept in out-patient treatment until an in-patient bed was available. What about the teen and the teen's family? What about the potential loss of life, a very real possibility for this particular individual?

Here was a staff member who desperately wanted to pour herself into her work and was blocked by rigid policies. Believe in your program and your personnel. Give them space to be creative; listen to their recommendations; make sure you are not blocking them because of your own fears and prejudices.

Once the directors hire the proper staff, orient them, and trust them, it becomes the practitioner's responsibility to honor the trust. For now the relationship between therapist and patient can determine the whole course of treatment for adolescents. True, young addicts can never get well until they want to and usually they do not want to until hitting "bottom." But in dealing with teens, we have to induce or invoke a "bottom" through education and therapy. First, we must get them to listen to us.

Some guidelines for staff who work with teens are:

Do not be a parent or a jailer with adolescents

If you talk down to them, they will ignore you and play your game. As soon as treatment is over, they'll do what they want, never having heard you. They need you to help them negotiate with the adult world in which they have to recover.

In addition, if you treat them with respect, as a fellow adult, they will probably try to live up to the new status. Ask them to help set treatment goals. They cannot work on everything in forty-five days, so let them pick out what they want to learn from you (solutions to sexual problems, dysfunctional families, abusive siblings, low self-esteem, propensity for failure). If they help design their therapy, they are more likely to respond to it.

Do not equate sobriety with traits and behaviors

Linda Yoakem describes another problem for us:

> Many adolescents get the message that even after they get clean and sober, they are not an okay person unless they cut their hair, change their clothing style, quit listening to heavy metal music, or otherwise change their appearance or tastes.

It is not wise to equate sobriety with traits and behaviors that do not relate to the disease. Holding up middle class America as the role model does not guarantee sobriety. Just as the disease has no respect for age, religion, cultural status, finances, or race, neither has recovery. Any questioning teenager is going to figure that out. Do not allow teens to shut you out because of your own biases. Amy, of Littleton, Colorado, said:

> Through my treatment, many counselors tried to convince me that my addiction was caused by certain music, posters, people and style of clothing. Well, I've learned myself that sobriety has little to do with objective surroundings, that I am staying sober for myself and because I want to.

Socializing with the client gives the message they are an okay person

Many treatment facilities believe that you must not socialize with your patients. George C. from Los Angles, California talked of the corporate structure he worked for:

> Certain treatment facilities in the country have the staff sign affidavits stating they will not have social relationships with patients up to two years after the patient leaves treatment or staff leaves employment of the facility.

I never could understand this. I can understand prohibiting sexual relationships because of the implied imbalance of power between patient and therapist. But the rule is simple. Do not have sex with your patients. If someone is so unethical that they will have sex with a patient, a contract is not going to stop them. As far as anything else, how can you tell a patient, "You're a good person. I like you. You are worth something," then turn around and say, "But I can't have anything to do with you outside of treatment." The subtle message is that they are not good enough to warrant friendship out of treatment.

Young people that I have worked with respond very well to seeing their therapists "on the outside." They socialize at AA, NA, and CA meetings and are very proud to know "respectable" people in their recovery. If clients are invited to their therapist's home for parties or dinners, they are thrilled. This gives clients the message that they are okay.

Do not give double messages

Another double message concerns personal lifestyles. If you cannot live the life you are asking your patients to live, then you should not be in the business.

Jim Balazs from Aurora, Colorado, shares his disappointment in the staff where he was treated:

> I helped the director of my residential treatment program move belongings after his apartment burned. I lost faith in people in general upon finding pot seeds and booze in his cupboards. Then my personal counselor took me out bowling the day after I graduated from thirteen months of treatment. Another counselor showed up drunk with two girlfriends who were also drunk. Great role models.

Believe in the disease concept

Believe the kids are really sick and they will believe it too. But if you minimize the problem, or "protect" patients from the truth, they'll go out and use again. One of the best stories to illustrate this comes from Perla P. of Colorado Springs, Colorado who is now twenty:

> Greg, age eighteen, Miles, age twenty-two, Linda, age eighteen, and I at fifteen went through treatment together five years ago and are still sober today. Very few others have stayed sober after going through this treatment center. Very few young people stay sober for more than a year or so in the community we live in.
>
> The two other guys that went through treatment with me, who stayed sober, and I have kept in close contact. We have talked with one another about the reasons we think we are still sober and so many others are not. We all agree that a great amount is attributed to the fact that while we were there, two men came to the treatment center twice a week and held a Step Study meeting. One of them had eleven years of sobriety and the other had eight. They gave each of us a step study format and gave us a new assignment to write about a step each week.
>
> They treated us as if we really were alcoholics who really had a disease that needed serious treatment. The steps were the treatment these two men had to offer. They also had a keen ability to catch us in our con games and they would not accept any horseplay from us.
>
> As a young person with only three years of actively abusing drugs and alcohol, I did not have much experience to compare myself to other recovering drunks. I remember asking one of these guys one day if I really was an alcoholic. He said "Yes." I feel that was very important to my young mind, to have an older "real alcoholic" confirm that I was also a "real alcoholic." Maybe the others that went through treatment with me and stayed sober had similar experiences.
>
> Maybe, however, the one most powerful thing we were given that others weren't was two alcoholic men who believed we had a deadly disease. Who also believed in the power of the steps because they had experienced the healing effects of this process themselves.

Deal with what you know

Do not take on a single problem that you know nothing or little about. You can't possibly be an expert in every aspect of your patient's life. These could include incest, sexual assault, child abuse (either to or by your patient) or depression. If their problems are beyond your scope, refer them to experts.

Experts are advancing a lot of theories right now about dysfunctional families and alcoholism, but do not be enamored by them. Incest, rape, child abuse, battering or other forms of abuse do not cause addiction. They may indeed be issues that have to be resolved for your patients, but the patient has to get clean and sober before being able to deal with much else. It may, and usually does, take years. Do not lead young people to believe that dealing with these issues will be sufficient to keep them sober. It will not. Furthermore, that belief can be a good excuse to keep using chemicals for years.

Working With Punks

Finally, let us discuss the tough, belligerent kids who drive you crazy. They are called punks. They will be your greatest challenge in treatment. They will be your greatest joy if you get through to them.

Establishing a productive therapeutic relationship is usually the largest stumbling block in working with punks. These kids do not trust and are almost phobic about acknowledging vulnerability. The stronger their image, the stronger the feelings underneath.

Mickie Moran, director of Rockford Memorial Outpatient in Rockford, Illinois designed some guidelines—The following suggestions are based primarily on her work.

DO

Understand why they are punks. Being a punk is a lot of work. You basically have to fight the entire adult world. You do not do it without a good reason. If you do not know the reason, your task should be to find out.

Be honest with them and be yourself. They are pros at spotting insincerity.

Know what they show and what they feel aren't usually the same and are often opposites (such as, "I don't care" = "I care too much." "I hate you" = "I trusted you and now it seems like you don't care about me.")

Stand up for them. They interpret loyalty as caring. If you are not willing to stand up for them, they do not think you care.

Set limits. Strength impresses them, gets their attention. Pick limits that have to do with their taking care of themselves, *not* limits that have to do with "rules and regulations." For example: "If you don't take a shower today, I'm going to recommend you eat in your room alone and do assignments alone. It's not okay with me that you don't take care of yourself and turn others off." instead of "I don't want to hear about you swearing in the waiting room again."

Make sure you follow through with what you say you are going to do. The secret here is to not back yourself into a corner. If you say you're going to isolate him if he does not wash again, make sure you really want to do that. Also think before you set up conditions. Punks are notorious at getting adults to threaten stupid things out of frustration. For example: "If you're late for one more activity, I'm going to discharge you."

Acknowledge their strengths. Punks tend to be very honest (emotionally honest, not always "fact" honest). They have a lot of integrity, but you have to know the game because they play by their rules, not yours. They usually stand up for underdogs and have a lot of guts. Once you get past the initial defiance, there is usually a lot of sensitivity and a good sense of humor.

Help establish reality testing. "Yep, the world really is unfair. How come you keep screwing yourself over trying to prove that it shouldn't be?"

Nurture them. Take interest in their hair and clothes, poetry, other things. Begin touching—holding hands, hugs. Do not go too fast with physical touch, especially if you know about or suspect a history of abuse.

Know they usually judge themselves more harshly than others do and have often decided they are hopeless "screw ups" or losers that will never amount to anything. Fears of being "crazy" or "bad" are common.

Give new views for old ideas. For example: "You're really a strong person to deal with how you feel," versus "Only wimps cry."

Use humor, especially paradoxical humor to confront. For example: "Look, if you're going to keep lying about this stuff, you've got to practice more. You can't even lie with a straight face. Why don't you try practicing with a mirror?"

Admit mistakes, especially when you feel like you blew it with them. You will be more real to them. You will also set a better example, build their trust, and you cannot fool them, anyway.

DON'T

Don't react out of your own stuff. The only way to avoid this is to be aware of what sets you off with adolescents in general and punks in particular. Most reactions come from fear. Punks are particularly adept at getting adults to react and are probably much more experienced at these kinds of battles than you are. Know your own attitudes about sex, criminal activities and bullies. If you are clear on your own feelings, punks will not be able to "trigger" your bad reactions. You know how you feel and can explain it without threatening or judging them. Instead of "Nobody's impressed, Big Shot," try "I don't think it's right to get your way with a switch blade because I don't believe anyone deserves to be terrorized. Besides it shows your weakness if you have to use a knife to get your way."

Don't get into power struggles with them. Setting limits is not a power struggle. You set the limits because you do not want them to hurt themselves or someone else. In a power struggle, you want to win and you want the kid to lose. For example: There is the "someone needs to teach that little asshole a lesson" mentality. If you get into a power struggle with a punk, you've already lost, at least therapeutically.

Don't buy their "it's everyone else's fault and they are all out to get me because they don't like long hair and leather" routine. Do not discount, though, their scapegoat role in the family, if it exists. Their families may be genuinely unreasonable with him or her.

Don't take their defiance at face value. Often it is a cover for other stuff— especially fear, sometimes shame or hurt. For example, "I'm not going to that bullshit reading group" may mean, "I don't know how to read and I'm afraid if I tell anyone, they'll make fun of me."

Don't believe their excuses. You do not have to push for change, but let them know you know it is crap.

Don't ignore their testing of limits (they will escalate the tests) or back down from them (they do not respect "suckers").

Don't accept their statements "You're the only one who understands me." It either diminishes them by making you responsible for developing the relationship, or it is a con.

Don't act like a parent and scold. Besides being offensive, it does not work.

Don't minimize feelings of "love" they have for another teenager or loyalty to their friends. These feelings are very intense for them and occupy most of their unstructured thought time.

Don't underestimate abandonment, separation, or grief issues, especially in regard to vacations, termination of treatment, transfer of therapist, etc. Punks are notorious for regression at the end of treatment to avoid saying goodbye.

Don't expect them to verbalize feelings other than anger right away. Remember their fear: the more afraid they are, the less safe it is for them to say so.

Chapter Highlights

1. When directors hire staff, they should hire people whose expertise is in the field of chemical addictions. In the treatment approach, focus on the addiction not the age of the patient.

2. Directors need to hire staff they believe in so they can give them the space to be innovative. They cannot let their own fears of corporate policy block good therapy practices. Success speaks for itself and corporate policy will always support successful treatment.

3. The relationship between patient and therapist can determine the whole course of treatment for the adolescent. Follow the hints and study the section, "Working with Punks."

Section III
Aftercare/Lifelines

Introduction

Even though programs in the field of chemical dependency often give the least amount of planning and energy to aftercare, this is the time that separates the heavyweight from the lightweight programs. It is relatively easy to keep patients drug free during treatment and next to impossible once they leave the treatment environment.

Once they leave the treatment center, adolescents must face all the obstacles they were shielded from while in treatment. This includes their friends who are still using, an unsympathetic school atmosphere, a home atmosphere that is adjusting at best and abusive at worst, and they must face free time without the supportive confines of treatment. The scary feelings of a whole new lifestyle must be confronted if they are to remain clean.

Aftercare is a transitional phase in recovery. It is not out-patient treatment. We assume that treatment has been given in the most responsible manner possible and aftercare is the phase in which treatment helps patients to apply what they have learned.

Aftercare is where we have decided what living conditions may best suit the recovery process for the adolescent. Do they go back home, or do they go to an institution, to a "safe" home, a long term half-way house? Or should we arrange emancipation?

Aftercare is where we help them adjust to school, new friends, and activities, and where we funnel them into a Twelve Step program for continuing abstinence. Aftercare is where we keep reminding young people about what they have already learned. Aftercare is crucial to the recovery process, in fact, it is the recovery process.

Yet most programs put very little energy into this important process. Motivation and education are the goal of in-patient treatment and a lifetime of sobriety is the goal of aftercare. Once adolescents leave treatment, recovery truly begins. In the world in which they will be required to live, drug free, they need the best aftercare help our centers have to offer.

Chapter 8

Aftercare

Aftercare, the most important part of staying clean following treatment, is often given the least attention by in-patient centers. It is usually a group for adolescents and parents who meet once a week to "discuss how the week has gone." This type of aftercare does not even begin to address the many issues that now face the newly sober teen. An aftercare that stops at one discussion group a week is wholly inadequate to help patients.

However, any aftercare program will not be able to keep patients and their families coming for long, no matter how good or bad the group's meetings. There are two good reasons for this:

     a) If the teen fails and begins using again, he will drop out, followed quickly by his parents.

     b) If the adolescent does very well and embraces a Twelve Step program of sobriety, he or she will be so busy getting well and being with new sober companions the new lifestyle will replace the group.

Either way aftercare, however important, will seldom last long. Therefore aftercare programs should be intense and condensed in order to fulfill the obligations they must meet. Instead of one group a week for a specified number of weeks, I would suggest a more accelerated approach. Four meetings a week for the first two weeks, then two meetings a week for two weeks, then (if you still have them coming) one a week for two weeks. That gives you fourteen meetings in six weeks, although you probably will not keep your patients for that length of time once treatment has ceased.

These fourteen meetings should include more than "discussions on how the week has gone." They should provide peer support, one-on-one counseling, emphasis on practicing principles within the family structure, and a support group for parents.

The program directors and therapists for aftercare have grave responsibilities to their patients. The fact that most centers give little attention to aftercare groups (except to say they have one) can be good news or bad. If therapists are bored with their job and feel "stuck" in a dead-end position, then it is bad news. However, if they like space and freedom, they can be very creative and innovative without the corporation breathing down their necks. The lack of structure does not have to be a negative feature of aftercare programs.

Be eclectic with this freedom. Know what your community has to offer for your sober teens and their parents and urge them into it whether it be ALANON, Alateen, ACOA, AA, NA, CA, PDAP (Twelve Step programs are described in Chapter 9), Tough Love groups, church programs, Outward Bound, or School Assistance Programs (SAPs). Draw heavily on volunteers. These are the institutions, support groups and people that your patients will have to rely on for a lifetime of support.

Funnel your patients to the right places and right people just as fast as you can. Do not believe that they will stay in your aftercare for long. They will not. Do not think that your hospital aftercare will work as a long-term program of sobriety.

Locating the right groups, bringing in volunteers, and getting teens the right sponsors in AA are not an abdication of your role. Become a "gateway therapist." Assess your patient's needs and funnel them in the community. You know that you and your program cannot be all things to all patients, but you can guide each teenager and parent to what they need.

You must get to know your AA, NA, CA, and PDAP communities. You have to develop a list of sponsors and court them. They will be the driving force in the teen's on-going recovery. That's reality. One of the aftercare therapist's responsibilities is to convince teens (if treatment already has not) that they cannot go it alone. They need a home group in AA (or other Twelve Step program) and they need a sponsor to teach them how sobriety works. If the client thinks he or she does not need a sponsor because they can do it their own way, the therapist must try to convince him or her otherwise. Char-Lee Dee, a Native American who has worked in NA for nineteen years, refers to kids doing it their own way as trying *designer recovery*. He says:

> Designer recovery. Doing it your own way. When you say things like, "I don't want to hear that. That's not what I need. I don't have to read that stuff. I don't need that step." My recommendation to them is this: Contact a trusted servant in NA World Services, Van Nuys, CA and ask them for an interview for the position of program redesigner. Don't accept less then $25,000. Get off your ass and into the Book!

When finding sponsors and groups for your adolescent patients, remember to utilize unusual people (see Chapter 7, Hiring Staff). People like Char-Lee really impress teenagers. He works well with them. They respond to his size and the fact that he is a minority. Teenagers believe this man will surely understand them.

"Biker" sober groups are a source of strength for adolescents, especially punks. They like the idea that tough, bad guys (and gals) are taking an interest in them. In Colorado Springs, the Serenity Riders offered to "host" a meeting at the local correctional facility. Personnel immediately panicked and limited the meeting to include only four sober bikers. The staff felt that the bikers were intimidating the kids. But Susan P., in charge of the bikers, said:

> The staff were the ones intimidated. They felt we were a security problem. But the kids really liked us. I feel that is because we speak the same language and are not afraid to swear. They can make a personal connection with us that they can't with a three-piece suit. With the suit you tend to think you can't have fun. But we can show them they can wear all this leather, stay sober, and have fun, too.

Not just Native Americans and bikers are good bets for adolescents—old timers can be gold mines when it comes to working with teens. They know sobriety and their years on Planet Earth have taught them a thing or two. Jim Ryan (sober forty-two years) works with kids all the time. He attributes his success (and believe me he has success) to his constant prayer asking God to put the right words in his mouth. He shares:

> I take them kids and hold their hands and let them shake. I talk about anything and everything until they stop shaking. Then I tell them about my disease. I was working with Cindy. I was fifty-eight and she was nineteen. "I'm different," she told me. I turned over my palm and said, "Me, too. See my fingerprints are different from yours and everyone else's." "No, I'm Indian," Cindy persisted. "Well, I'm Irish and it didn't have a damned thing to do with it. We're both God's children aren't we?" That broke the ice. I always pray I'll say the right words and that the Good Lord puts them there. Cindy's whole body was trembling with fright. The kid's do not know what love is so you have to show them. I said, "Cindy, put your arms around me and say I love you." She put her arms around me and I said, "This is God's Love." Cindy is now sober thirteen years.

Volunteers are your backbone. Use them. Bring them to your kids and send your kids to them. Learning your community's resources with a few months of footwork can make or break your aftercare program.

Aftercare will actually begin while the teenager is still in treatment. The aftercare therapist will be in close contact with the primary in-patient counselor. Together they will decide where the patient's needs are best met: home, a safe home, emancipation, or another alternative (see Chapter 9, Going Back Home). Then the aftercare group should help the patient deal with the post-treatment plan.

David Marvin, aftercare coordinator of New Beginnings in Denver, says:

> It's really a stacked deck against kids because of where they are in maturation. They think they are invincible. It's hard for them to realize they have an incurable disease for the rest of their life. In aftercare I have to help them adjust to that and keep reminding them of something that is so hard for them to believe.
>
> Our group is a working support group. Generally they are with other people they've met in treatment and with their parents. They're working on things they've established in their home contracts. This is an attempt to continue to work on family communications, peer support, and parental peer support.

Although I do not personally believe in home contracts, because contracts are only made to be broken, it does make clear the expectations between adolescent and parent. It gives the family a document from which to work. It gives the aftercare group a basis from which to begin "work" on the family dynamics. If your center chooses to make contracts, understand that the document has nothing to do with the kid's sobriety, it only has to do with family expectations. Again, contracts, a behaviorist's tool, designed to treat behavior problems; they are not a framework from which to stay clean and sober.

Probably the most important function of aftercare is to help prevent relapse while teenagers struggle with a new lifestyle. Not only does their disease impel them to use drugs again, not only do their old drug friends push for them to use again, but the prejudices against their youth push, too.

The younger you are when you get sober, the harder people will try to convince you as you get older that you do not suffer from any addictive disease.

Adolescents have to be prepared for this pressure. It is a lot harder to deal with than we think. The main reason for this difficulty is that the disease is always lurking under the surface, trying to gain an active foothold again. As therapists, we should concern ourselves with this very real jeopardy for teenage alcoholic/addicts. If enough people frequently tell them they are not sick, at some point in sobriety they may succumb. Teddy, sixteen years old, was told, "You're too young to be an alcoholic." "Oh yeah," she'd reply, "can you guarantee me I'll live long enough to become old enough?" That is the only answer that makes sense.

When we speak of the possible causes of relapse we have to:

Make them aware of the symptoms of relapse

Identify the high risk situations

Present an alternative behavior for them to use

Warning Signs Of Relapse In The Adolescent

Supersensitivity to everything. They begin to take anything you say as an insult. "Why does everyone keep singling me out?"

Self-pity and boredom. They begin to whine and complain of nothing to do. They get into the "poor me" stuff. "No one really likes me at school, not even my teachers."

Depression and isolation. They stop sharing feelings and start living inside themselves instead of outside. They suddenly prefer not to participate in family, peer, or Twelve Step activities.

Confusion. Irrational thinking begins. They blame others unjustly for their troubles. They do not see their own responsibility in matters. "My alarm didn't go off so I'm late. It wasn't my fault."

Physical restlessness. They begin to display agitation, shaky hands. They may not be able to sit still for class, therapy, meetings, or TV.

Anger and resentment. Possible explosive behavior. They now do not like what parents, therapists, or sober friends say. "That doesn't apply to me because ...." They ascribe to "designer recovery" at this point.

Big deals. Everything now takes on overwhelming proportions. A cut finger is surely blood poisoning. A failed test is grounds for quitting school. A quarrel with a friend means they'll never speak to each other again.

Faulty memory. They begin to remember all the good times drinking and drugging and not the bad times. "I'm missing all the fun. Going to parties doesn't hurt anyone."

Everyone's an enemy. They get into the "us against them" stuff with all authority figures. They're fighting a private war with the world. "There's no point in getting a license because they'll never let me have a car, anyway."

Withdraws from sober support. They shun their school support group, drop their sponsor, and quit attending meetings. At this point, the teenager believes (however falsely) that he can spend time with old drugging friends and "handle" things.

Identifying High Risk Behaviors

This sounds easy but for the adolescent it is not. Remember, adolescents believe they are invincible. They always believe they can handle more than they actually can. Therefore, in groups we must impress upon them our frailties as humans and the power of the disease. They must learn that everyone, not just teens, must shield themselves from high risk behaviors which include:

Maintaining friendships with old drug friends is the most dangerous high risk behavior, almost insuring a relapse.

Going to parties where drugs and booze are served.

Staying in enclosed areas where people smoke pot (like cars and bathrooms).

Constant fighting with boyfriends and girlfriends or family members (see number 4 of Symptoms Leading to Relapse).

Going to bars or head shops.

Accompanying "friends" or family on drug runs.

High risk behaviors are not limited to this list, but these are some of the most significant ones.

A Tae Kwan Do master explains, "the best way to win a fight is not to be there." Thus, we are asking teenagers to win the fight by not being there. So where should they be?

Alternative Activities

In AA, members will learn to call their sponsors or clean and sober friends, go to meetings, read their literature, and work their steps. All these things will help arrest their disease. But what about spare time?

Aftercare can help organize sober social functions. It is a very positive approach and something more than "discussing the way the week went." When teenagers stay clean and sober, they love opportunities to participate in sober activities with other sober people. Mike C., from Littleton, says:

> I'm more happy and more like a kid than I've ever been. Since starting my recovery I've done more childish things than ever, and I love it.

Mike will never regain his childhood or innocence, but he is now able to let the child in him enjoy sober activities. I observed Mike, age sixteen, organizing a sledding trip to the mountains. The other kids in his aftercare group got very excited. One boy even decided to take the day off work so he could go with the rest of them. I loved watching the enthusiasm. Camille, age sixteen (sober two years), from Denver shares:

> When I was using, I was a "childish adult." When I started to recover, I became an adult trying to develop my child-like qualities.

Again, the innovativeness of the professional is the crux of the treatment program. Lousy staff, lousy program. Creative staff, creative sobriety. David Moran from New Beginnings likes to encourage his teen patients to go to Outward Bound, where outdoor skills are honed and they gain a new-found confidence in their ability to deal with the world and other people.

Camille, from Denver, shared with me one thing she does as an alternative behavior to using. She writes sober poems. Then she contrasts them to her using poems.

> I wrote *The Rain* in my last days of using. It always seemed that I was tense and my emotions felt heavy. Somehow I was able to cry and get a bit of relief from this "ache." It's not nearly as emotional as the releases I have today. It was kind of like okay to take this heaviness off my shoulders.

THE RAIN

The rain to me represents the emotions in my head.
The tension in the air before the gray clouds burst their
Rain drops, equals the tension
In my soul before my eyes release their oceans of tears.
The pounding, burning heat on the pavement reminds me of
The heat my flushed skin feels after the abuse you push towards me
Then the pitter patter of the rain cools off the heated ground.
Just like my tears cool down my heated temper.
Then the rain leaves and everything
Is clean and fresh, just like
My tears dry and my torment is drained.
But then the heat builds along with the tension in the air.
And again my emotions thunder
In my head and the tension is again in my soul.

This next poem was one of the first times in my sobriety that I experienced true joy and happiness. It hit me and I didn't know what was happening. I realized that I was ecstatic for no real reason except life itself and I burst into tears.

GOD FOUND

The clouds are clearing
The rainbows appearing
The thunder is quieting
The faces are smiling
The wind is calming
The weather is balmy
Living's not fighting.
The sun is shining
What I have now I do not want to lose.
I have a choice and it's this life I choose
Being here now is so happy and exciting
Living in peace without all of that fighting.
Sad times are easier, bad times are all right
Having friends like you, with whom I am tight.
Knowing that all this can come to an end
Striving to keep what I have so I'll win.

Every time I feel like using, I look at the last few poems I wrote before I sobered up and I know there's no way I can go back to that.

Aftercare—the beginning of life!

Chapter Highlights

1. Become a "gateway therapist" by funnelling your patients to the right people and meetings needed to maintain sobriety. Do not think they will stick with aftercare for long. They will not.

2. Helping prevent relapse is a major goal of aftercare. Help teens recognize relapse, identify high risk behavior, and develop alternative behaviors.

3. Each treatment center should consider sponsoring sober activities for their graduates. These could be dances, ski trips, swimming parties, camp outs—anything kids would enjoy doing clean and sober.

Resources

Periodicals

Knoll, Scotte. 1988 "Meeting Special Needs: A Holistic Approach to Chemical Abuse," *Student Assistance Journal*, Nov/Dec.

Chapter 9

Going Back Home

Although treatment offers isolation and hope to stay sober, the struggle of reality only starts when the isolation ends.

Amy F.

It is now time to organize the parents and their children and implement certain plans. These plans naturally begin while your patient is still in treatment. Although the plans for going home will be developed among the treatment staff, parents, and adolescent patient, most of the responsibility should be given to the adolescent to determine what he or she feels would be the safest environment to return to.

The options vary, with some "better" choices and choices mandated by circumstances. The most desirable option is for the adolescent to return to the primary home with a family interested in his or her recovery offering love and support. But the best choices may not be possible, so be prepared to explore alternatives.

Safe Homes

Safe homes are alternative homes that some adolescents must be placed in because it is not safe to return to their primary home. There may be multiple reasons for this. Possibly there were violence and physical abuse by either or both parents. Incest issues may make it impossible for the patient to return. Sometimes one or both parents are themselves alcoholic/addicts. Maybe they just smoke pot, but it is too uncomfortable for the recovering teen. Sometimes the adolescent lives in a home that is not near a school with a strong support group, and it is impossible for the core family to move. Whatever the reason, there are several types of "safe" homes to examine.

The first type of safe home placement is with a relative or close friend who wants to help. Occasionally this means going to live with the non-custodial parent if the original parents are separated or divorced. Recovering adolescents could live with a grandparent, aunt, uncle, or close friend of the family. Make sure that if one of these alternatives is chosen, the surrogate parents are educated about enabling and understand what is expected for the patient's aftercare.

In some cases the state takes over and places the teen in a foster home. Although this is one of the least desirable locations for a recovering teen, under some circumstances it may be the only viable choice. In some states, however, welfare systems have begun a new foster home program called "Sober Safe Homes."

A Sober Safe Home is a licensed foster care home in which either one or both adults are clean and sober in a Twelve Step program. Most often, the couple does not accept money for this but helps a recovering child as a part of their personal Twelve Step for recovering adults. If there is not a system like this set up in your community, it is worth having your outreach worker get some Sober Safe Homes licensed so they are an available option in your aftercare program.

There are obvious advantages to a Sober Safe Home as compared to regular foster care. One is that the state or parents usually don't have to pay, although they can. But more important is that the recovering young adult will get the guidance and support of an AA environment. Other than returning to a loving family, this is the best choice for most recovering teens.

Emancipation

Another choice upon leaving treatment is emancipation. Most states have provisions for emancipating kids over the age of sixteen if they can show they are capable of caring for themselves. Many times the recovering teenagers I have encountered are perfectly capable of taking care of themselves—often they have been doing so for quite some time anyway. You may find that if your patient refuses to go home or back to school, you can help them with employment and help them start legal proceedings for emancipation. All outreach workers and aftercare therapists that work with adolescents should be familiar with procedures for emancipation.

Two For One

In Georgia and North Carolina, there are some Drug Action programs that are quite innovative. Centers are set up in large metropolitan areas for in-patient treatment. However kids are accepted from all over the state. Once the intensive in-patient treatment is finished, approximately a thirty day period, the aftercare begins. In aftercare, the patient is still required to be at the center every day after school and on weekends.

Obviously, this is not possible for the teens from out of town. To solve this problem, the Drug Action team came up with a remarkable solution. For families from the core treatment area, they put one teenager in treatment and take two home. The families from out of town pay a nominal fee to the families in town for room and board for their child.

For any child having to return to a community with little or no support in a program of recovery, this is an excellent solution. In addition, this can reinforce staying sober for both young adults coming out of treatment. Every treatment center ought to offer families the opportunity to participate in the "two for one" program. It can save rural patients from almost certain relapse and it can strengthen the peer support of the host family's child. Again, this is something for your outreach worker or aftercare therapist to set up.

Halfway House Or Long-Term Treatment

Sometimes a much stronger support is needed initially. In general, I do not support long-term treatment (over several months) when the patient begins recovery. It seems ludicrous to keep young adults in actual treatment at hospital prices past the education/motivation phase unless they have severe psychiatric problems. However a half-way house with other recovering young people and adults can be conducive to recovery. Kevin O., sober four years from age seventeen, shares:

> I wasn't welcome home following treatment at Cottonwood unless I went to a half-way house for ninety days. I was given the opportunity to grow partly because my family gave me the room. I also had to find the willingness from a Power greater than myself. The halfway house gave me the opportunity to gradually get (for the first time) into the mainstream of life. I didn't really know what it was like to be sober in the real world.

In deciding which of the above options is best for your patients, let them understand that you know the difficulties inherent in growing up and getting sober at the same time. Let them know you are concerned about their goals, family, school, peer problems and recovering life in general. Perhaps the main point to emphasize is that no matter where they live, recovery is the hardest, most difficult thing they will ever have to do. Their living situation may make it easier, but it is never easy to live through the process of recovery.

As Mike C. from Littleton, Colorado, says:

> Often you have gone through treatment and you get out. Things are going well, then something from the past gets you: legal troubles, like me facing jail, or old family problems. You must remember why you got sober. It was for you. No one else but yourself.

There are three main points to be absolutely firm on when it is time to send teens home.

Do not send kids home to any environment where school support is minimal or nonexistent, or when there is little Twelve Step support. A home community must have an AA or NA club, at least one young people's meeting a week, a Twelve Step meeting everyday, and/or PDAP support. If the community does not meet these requirements, the chances of the patient's staying clean and sober are practically nil. Be absolutely clear on this matter with the patient and the parents while discussing alternative living situations if the need arises.

Under no circumstances allow a child to return to a physically or sexually abusive home. If it requires legal action to keep them from going home, take it. No young adult can even think about staying clean and sober if he or she is being beaten up or involved in an incestuous relationship.

If there is booze, marijuana, or prescription drugs at home that make your patients uncomfortable, do not let them go home until these items are removed. They are going to have a rough time without being tempted when they grab an apple next to the beer in the refrigerator, or see diet pills beside their toothbrush, or have to smell pot when they come home from school. George C., from California, says:

> I told my father to remove the booze from the house, that it would make my sobriety less prone to temptation.

And Camille, from Denver, shares:

> On my first pass I asked a family member to remove the liquor from our home or I would not come home. I feel that it's my responsibility to do whatever I need to do if a situation is threatening my sobriety.

Back To School

Going back to school is an important aspect of the adolescents' recovery. Here they will face the worst possible environment for staying clean and sober. They will be right in the midst of their using friends, the pressure to belong and be liked, the pressure of "us against them" leading to "let's get stoned, Dude."

If a student expresses fear about returning to the same school, do not minimize his objections. It may in fact be best that he does not return to that pressure. Peer pressure is very real and more intense than we can possibly imagine. No one should be expected to stay clean when constantly offered drugs and alcohol. If patients say "no" to their old school, it is our responsibility to work out something more appropriate for them.

Another reason for not sending teens back to their old school is that the system may not have adequate support for recovering teens. Do not confuse alcoholism education, "Just Say No" programs, counseling, or awareness programs with support groups for recovering alcoholic/addicts. Most high schools have education and support programs for students who do not want to use. There are campaigns for sober teen taxi services and Prom Promises where students swear not to use alcohol and drugs one particular night. But remember, a support group for kids who do not want to use is not the same as a support group for abstinent addicts. If the patient's school does not have a peer support group for recovering alcoholic/addicts, do not send him or her back.

These support groups can be of several different types but should always meet during school hours. There are too many reasons students might not be able to meet after school. These reasons could include school sports activities, after school jobs, or younger siblings at home whom the teen must watch. Although not everyone at the schools can be experts on the disease, staff must give their students the opportunity for support during recovery. The Board of Education policy for the school district of Beloit, Wisconsin, has a realistic attitude:

> The greatest responsibility for dealing with chemical abuse rests with the student and his or her parents, but the school has a legitimate concern when school performance is affected. It is, therefore, the policy of the School District of Beloit to deal with such problems as follows:
>
> The School District recognizes that many student problems can be successfully treated, especially if they are identified in the early stages and an appropriate referral is made. (See Chapter 1 Identifying the Troubled Teen.)
>
> The purpose of this policy is to assure students that if personal problems are the cause of unsatisfactory school performance, they will receive consideration and assistance in seeking help to resolve such problems.

This SAP (School Assistance Program) goes on to explain that counseling is available for students who feel they need it and support is given to students returning from treatment. This is minimal involvement but still quite adequate as long as the schools offer support in the form of recovering peer groups.

At Palisades High in California, the school psychologist, Linda Levine, helped start an AA group. It meets once a week during lunch and remains anonymous, according to AA tradition. School officials or parents are not informed of the names of participants and Dr. Levine's only duty is to open the door to the meeting room.

Other schools have recovery support groups that alternate between different class periods each week. This way, the students do not miss too much of any single class and can be excused for that one class every six weeks. Mike C., from Littleton, Colorado says:

> My school has a terrific aftercare type group. We meet once a week. Each week we alternate periods, and we discuss how we're feeling and problems we're having.

Camille's been going to her school support group for two years:

> Our school has a support group that meets on Tuesdays on different periods every week. We stay away from the AA and NA name because it's a group lead by the social worker or counselor. Twelve Step meetings are not therapy groups.

Some school systems have highly developed SAPs for alcoholics returning to school. Of course, the more intense the program, the more likely your patient will remain sober. More prevalent, however, are schools with one or two staff members trained to help in chemical dependency problems, offering some education and hopefully, a sober support group.

In Anchorage, the school system and programs designed to help recovering youth have created a remarkable support plan. All the teens returning from treatment enroll in the same school regardless of where they live. Parents and school personnel make sure that recovering students have transportation to school. Hopefully, other school districts will follow their lead. This is the type of SAP program that really aids students in recovery. The peer pressure is then used in a positive, rather then negative, manner.

If it is clear that your patient should not return to his or her old school because of reasonable objections or because of inadequate school support, there are alternatives:

> Night school, where the peer pressure might not be as intense and most work is done at home in a safer environment.

Home schooling with a tutor or parent. Many states have provisions for this and it is a viable option as long as the teen can stay involved with kids in AA, NA, CA, or PDAP so that they are not isolated.

Alternative schooling is now offered in many areas where "difficult" or pregnant students can go. Education at these locations is more individually tailored to student's needs.

After age sixteen, students can acquire a GED then begin college or take a part time job.

You can arrange for your client to change schools to one that has a strong SAP in chemical dependency. Some parents are in a position to move. If not, explore the option of a host home.

Twelve Step Programs

The greatest obstacles to funnelling your young patients into AA, NA, and CA are the club house controversies and of a more serious nature, the "pure" alcoholic versus the drug addict controversy. Both of these issues must be addressed during treatment before the adolescent faces them in recovery.

AA and NA have, for years, had members open private clubs where sober people can meet, hold meetings, and sponsor other sober functions. Unlike AA, these clubs are private and can bar anyone who does not meet their clubhouse rules. Some will not allow drunk people in, some won't allow children running around, some disallow teenagers.

Teenagers have been barred from many clubs because of obnoxious behavior. Sometimes the culprits are not the recovering adolescents, but Alateens or various other kids hanging around using (or misusing) club facilities. In an old club in Denver, teenagers from a "home" across the street were hanging out, disrupting, and sexually acting out though they were not there for sobriety—just laughs. Naturally club members complained and finally had them barred.

In another clubhouse in Aurora, Colorado, some Alateens hung out, were rambunctious and disturbed the regular members. Their antics got so out of hand one day that a teen slung a pool ball which broke a plate glass window. This cost the members $1000 and created bad feelings about teens using their facilities.

Recovering teenagers, just like any recovering addicts, need sober places to congregate and socialize. They need the AA and NA clubs, which are private, dues-paying operations. The teens must be taught how to behave and why. Part of a teen's treatment program should include instruction on how to conduct oneself in this environment. Nancy B., receptionist at a club in Denver, relates the following story:

A youngster sauntered into the club and asked me, "Where's the meeting?" I told him, but it wasn't right then so I told him to go get a cup of coffee and wait for the meeting to start. He whipped through the club and came roaring back to me, "There's just a bunch of old people in here. Where's a place with kids?" To which I answered, "Listen kid, if you're an alcoholic, it doesn't make any difference how old *we* are." Does he want to get sober or play?

This adolescent may want to get sober. However, his attitude has not communicated this. A few simple guidelines presented in treatment will help.

Guidelines For Teens Using Twelve Step Clubs

No disruptive antics. Act responsibly and with respect toward your fellow recovering alcoholic/addicts. Laugh, have fun, socialize—save the animal behavior for outside so club members believe you are serious about sobriety.

Always pay dues. If you use the facility, support your club. Paying dues also gives you a say in how things are done. You always had money to use drugs, so you can pay your own way here. Just because you are young is no excuse to sponge off sober adults.

Never drag your using friends or siblings to clubs. If they want help, take them to treatment or a meeting. Unless friends are on a path to recovery, they should not be at these private clubs. People who are still using destroy the atmosphere by selling drugs, sexually acting out, smelling bad, looking bad, and acting bad. The other members do not need it.

Do not succumb to the reverse prejudice and subtly put recovering adults down. Do not act like you are somehow smarter because you got to AA sooner than they. Getting to AA at a younger age does not increase a person's stature in the group. In recovery, all are equal.

Camille from Denver, who is sixteen years old but first came to a
club at age fourteen, describes her experience:

> When I first came to an AA club, I was treated much differently. I
> was told that the club wasn't a teenage hangout. I accepted that and
> right away paid my dues, went to meetings, and displayed responsible,
> recovering behavior. I proved I wasn't going to dance on the tables or
> anything. Today I'm accepted, I'm finally one of them. I also have
> started a young people's meeting in this very club.

The second major controversy within the AA club houses is an
emotionally charged one—the "pure" alcoholics in AA versus all the
other addicts. As a prominent representative from a New York service
committee defines it:

> Alcoholism is different from other drug addictions in both the
> disease and lifestyle. We in AA would be shirking our responsibility to
> the alcoholic if we let in just any addict. We can't really help addicts
> because we "pure" alcoholics had a different life and do not relate.
> Therefore it isn't good for either of us to mix programs and meetings.
> Besides, AA was started just for alcoholics and that says it all.

But, alcoholism is addiction and the biological aspects of any drug
addiction are basically the same. AA describes alcoholism as a "mental
obsession coupled with a physical compulsion." This is the definition of
any addiction.

Young people need to learn this basic truth of addiction. An addict is
an addict is an addict. We cannot afford to separate the chemicals and
describe them as different diseases with different recoveries. Recovery is
the same. Bill Wilson in *Alcoholics Anonymous* clearly stated, "We
realize we know only a little. God will constantly disclose more to you
and to us." Nothing is written in concrete and this has to be stressed with
the young recovering people.

Bill Wilson, the first member of AA, was exclusively an alcoholic
and the second member, Bob, generalized to other drugs as well as
alcohol. They both knew you could not stop drinking while using other
drugs nor stop using drugs while drinking. The fact that AA stands for
"Alcoholics" only means that the founder of AA was struggling with the
drug alcohol. Addiction is the disease and alcohol is one chemical that
people become addicted to in our society. Bill's primary drug of choice

was alcohol, and thus we have AA. If it had been valium, we may have been joining "Valiums Victorious."

In any case, it is vitally important that newcomers to recovery from mind-affecting chemicals do not listen to the stilted, narrow objections some people may give them. Young people have access to many mind-affecting chemicals. Many of them will die thinking different chemicals cause different diseases. How many of them will try every chemical to find the magic one, like alcoholics used to switch drinks trying to control their disease? Chad, from Denver, shares:

> I gave up drugs with the help of alcohol and it was alcohol that got me to recovery. But it could have been the other way around. A drug is a drug. However, old timers sometimes do not acknowledge that because they stay sober on tranquilizers. It's not nice to say but true. So they do not want to hear a drug is a drug. They do not even want to hear that alcohol is a drug. I think that treatment centers need to inform patients that non-alcoholics, people whose primary addiction was something else may not be welcomed at closed meetings of AA.

This is true. They need to be informed. Forewarned is forearmed. And since this is the teens' lifeline, they need to consider whatever obstacles they might encounter and decide on a plan of action before they face these issues. Camille says:

> Yes, there's controversy in Twelve Step groups but if you want recovery, nothing as ridiculous as the controversy will keep you from recovery.

The crux of any adolescent's sobriety is successful entry into a Twelve Step program. Nothing else seems to effectively arrest the disease of addiction in adults and in younger members. With this observation, here is a brief evaluation of the programs that are the lifeline to teens.

Alcoholics Anonymous

AA is a group of men and women who meet and offer support to each other for sobriety from alcohol and other mind-affecting chemicals that interfere with that sobriety. They practice sound principles of living by following a Twelve Step program of recovery from the disease of alcoholism/addiction.

It is the "Mother" program of all the other Twelve Step programs and has the strongest outreach, with more members than any other recovery program in the world. As such, anyone in recovery should belong to at least one AA home group to insure a solid foundation in recovery.

The biggest obstacles for young people in The AA Program are those members that still feel kids are "too young" to have a serious problem and the "pure" alcoholics who believe no one can mention drugs in a meeting. Since 80 percent of all people now entering AA are multi-drug abusers/addicts who are beginning recovery at younger ages every year, the obstacles will eliminate themselves soon enough. In the meantime, young people can find meetings that do not make these distinctions (they exist all over, especially in the Young People's Meetings); they can ignore people with objections to how they introduce themselves or what chemical they refer to in their talks; or they can fight for change in service work.

Whatever your patients choose to do will depend on their personality. Amy F., from Littleton, Colorado, tells what she does:

> I've found in my recovery that I feel I can only go to certain AA meetings because of my age. I'm sick of hearing, "you're so lucky to only be nineteen." It doesn't matter what sex, race, or age one is. We all have one thing in common. We are addicts, whether the problem is drugs or alcohol.

Narcotics Anonymous

Narcotics Anonymous is based on the Twelve Steps of AA and run in the same manner. The main difference between AA and NA is that in the first step, NA addresses the disease and AA refers to the chemical. AA says "We were powerless over alcohol..." and NA says "We were powerless over our addiction..."

More "hard core" type addicts frequent NA meetings. Any of your patients that were street people, used needles, or dealt drugs would benefit greatly from the identification in NA. These people tend to "get down" and "tell it like it is." They are good at confronting and generally do not have a problem with the idea that teens under the age of twenty are just as sick as they are.

The only obstacle the young addict might encounter in NA is a type of reverse prejudice about AA. Since AA has made a stink about the "pure" alcoholics only talking in closed meetings, some NAs ask members not to introduce themselves as alcoholics. It's a silly controversy and should be given no more thought than the AA side of it.

Cocaine Anonymous

Again, this is like NA and, where available, would be very beneficial for those whose primary drug of choice is cocaine. I would not, however, advise anyone to go exclusively to CA but to supplement it with AA and NA for the support. CA as yet has not subscribed to the controversy that some AA and NA members seem to be caught up in and displays more of the loving tolerance that both AA and NA are built on.

Palmer Drug Abuse Program

From the PDAP stated purpose:

> PDAP is a two-part family program which offers help to both teenagers and adults who express a desire to find an alternative to drug and alcohol use, and to parents who seek solutions to family and personal conflicts arising from drug or alcohol use by a family member. Treatment is of a multi-disciplinary approach, involving evaluation and intervention, individual counseling, peer support and values clarification, and interpersonal drug-free recreation.

It is also a Twelve Step based program, although the steps have been slightly changed. PDAP is a great program for intact families, for teens who are simply abusers and want to stop using, and for those in the very early stages of the disease who have not had much trouble but have been identified as alcoholic/addicts either through genetics or lab tests.

Don't get me wrong. I am not saying it's a "wimp" program. PDAP has saved many lives and families and is very successful in its scope. But just as NA is for "hard core" addicts, PDAP is for "soft core" addicts or abusers. This is the program you could refer families to whose children are abusing but may not actually be addicts, or those in the very beginning states of disease who may not identify with full-blown addicts and alcoholics.

PDAP is not always appropriate. Lily B., now in Eagle Lodge in Denver, Colorado, had been court-ordered to PDAP at age fifteen. She shares:

> I liked it because it was for teens. They had dances. You could go there and hang out and play cards. I went to some meetings and I tuned them out. I thought most of those kids were full of shit. I had a real arrogant attitude. I was from the streets and these kids got caught stealing some of Dad's booze. Big deal. I didn't relate to them.
>
> I thought maybe I had a problem but I'd outgrow it. In any case, I wasn't like the PDAPers. They were pretty innocent.

Other Twelve Step Programs

Alanon, Alateen, ACOA and other related programs for the family are wonderful for interested family members. Do not send alcoholic/addicts to any related programs, even if they qualify, until they have over a year of sobriety. The chemically dependent person needs to pour every ounce of energy into recovery and not worry about the related problems of dysfunctional families or other alcoholic family members. Later they may very well need these related self-help programs, but not before their primary disease is well under control.

Summary

I will consider my research and this book a success if you receive no other messages than the following:

Adolescence is not the disease—alcoholism/addiction is. Treat the disease, not the developmental stage.

All alcoholics who began drinking in their teens, whether they're thirteen or fifty-three, will be at the emotional stage of a teen when they begin recovery.

Differences between treating an adolescent and adult are minimal, not unlike the minor differences in treating women, Blacks, Vietnamese, or the disabled.

The advantages of mainstreaming teenagers in treatment far outweigh the disadvantages.

Aftercare is the ultimate measure of a treatment program.

Chapter Highlights

1. There are numerous reasons why adolescents may or may not return home. Although their living situation is not responsible for recovery, some places are safer environments in which to live a program of sobriety. Under no circumstances let a child return to a physically or sexually abusive home.

2. An adolescent should only return to a school where the SAP program has a strong support group for recovering youth. If a school does not have a support program, teenagers should consider other alternatives for continuing their education.

3. Teenagers need to be taught how to behave in AA and NA clubs. The club atmosphere and socializing in the Twelve Step programs are their lifeline to a clean and sober lifestyle.

4. It is important to funnel adolescents into Twelve Step programs designed to treat addiction. The teenager should set aside the related family programs, Alanon, Alateen, ACOA until the primary disease is well under control. Then and only then should related programs be considered.

Resources

Books

Alcoholics Anonymous. NY: AA World Services, Inc., 1939.

Baron, Jason D., *The Parent's Handbook of Drug Abuse and Treatment.* Houston: DAPA, 1981.

Marshall, Shelly, *Young, Sober, & Free.* Center City, Minnesota: Hazelden, 1978.

Narcotics Anonymous. Van Nuys: NA World Services, Inc. 1982.

Periodicals

Kantrowitz, Barbara and Jeanne Gordon. 1988. "A New Course on Campus: AA 101." *Newsweek* Nov. 28: 63.

Knoll, Scotte. 1988. "Meeting Special Needs: Holistic Approach to Chemical Abuse." *Student Assistance Journal* Nov/Dec.

Appendix 1

Treatment Paternalism in Chemical Dependency Counselors

Michael J. Marshall, Ph.D., North Carolina A & T State University
Shelly Marshall, B.S., Youth Enjoying Sobriety Retreat
Key words: Adolescent alcoholism, alcoholism counselors, paternalism, medical model, recovered counselors
Requests for reprints should be sent to: Michael J. Marshall, Department of Psychology, North Carolina A & T State University, Greensboro, NC 27411.

Abstract

This study investigated the degree of paternalism in the treatment philosophies of chemical dependency counselors in three categories of treatment centers— adolescent-only, adult, and religious/minority. Counselors were shown picture arrays of either adolescent patients or adult patients and asked to choose a preferred treatment policy, either paternalistic or compensatory in nature. Results showed religious/minority counselors preferred a significantly greater paternalistic approach to all patients than did the adolescent-only and adult center counselors. The adolescent-only counselors responded more paternalistically to the adolescent patients than the adult patients, while the adult and religious/minority counselors did not respond significantly different to either group.

Treatment Paternalism in Chemical Dependency Counselors

In the past, few adolescent addict/alcoholics received treatment (Meacham, 1989). Those who did were primarily treated in adult clinics (Zimmermen, 1990) and "storefront" religious centers. But in the last ten years young addict/alcoholics have increasingly been treated in chemical dependency treatment programs that specialize in adolescents, with a resultant dramatic rise in the number of adolescent admissions (Darnton, 1989; Meacham, 1989; Zimmermen, 1990). Although many professionals assume the treatment outcome for adolescents is superior in adolescent-only treatment programs (Moorhouse,1989; Zimmerman, 1990), there exists a paucity of research that has addressed the relative efficacy of adult versus adolescent-oriented treatment, nor quantified differences in treatment structure, content, philosophy, and staff orientation.

Kazdin et al. (1990), a review of the adolescent psychotherapy research literature concluded that so few studies have been done on extended treatment in clinical settings for adolescents that any conclusions or assumptions about it are premature. The few studies that focused directly on adolescent in-patient addiction treatment analyzed family demographics, chemical use etiology, and resistence to treatment, rather than the therapists' attitudes (Taffaro & Forsyth, 1989; Piercy & Frankel, 1989; Needle et al., 1988). One study that did look at the therapists' attitudes and expectations in family therapy for drug addicts (although not limited to adolescents) concluded that the therapists' expectations undermined the patient's assumption of personal accountability and negatively affected recovery outcome (Reichelt & Christensen, 1990).

While numerous studies have examined adult post-treatment abstinence rates (Marlatt et al., 1988), few studies examined adolescent abstinence rates, possibly because adolescent treatment tends to focus upon substance dependence as more a symptom of interpersonal relationship problems rather than as a biological or psychological malfunction (Schwartz, 1989). Two of the studies located did not use complete abstinence as a criterion for success. One measured reduction in drug use prior to and at the end of treatment (Friedman et al., 1986) while the other used "abstinent/essentially abstinent," where a few weeks of using drugs after treatment was still considered successful (Alford et al., 1991). We found one study that claimed adolescent rates of abstinence at six months to be as high as 30 percent (Brown et al., 1989). Since the figure was derived from only 88 percent of the adolescents that could be found after treatment and interviews were done with parents escorting their children to the clinics, where parental disfavor could influence the adolescent to lie. The validity of Brown's results are questionable. Marlatt et al. (1988) concluded, after reviewing over 70 studies of chemical dependency outcomes, that fewer than 15 percent of subjects remained completely abstinent after treatment.

An appropriate classification scheme for chemical dependency treatment models is necessary in order to conceptualize the difference between the standard adult model of treatment, the newer adolescent-only treatment approach, and traditional religious solutions. Brickman et al. (1982) offer four general models that do a good job of differentiating the philosophies of these three common approaches to chemical dependency treatment.

In the first [*moral model*], actors are held responsible for both problems and solutions and are believed to need only proper motivation. In the *compensatory model*, people are seen as not responsible for problems but responsible for solutions, and are believed to need power. In the *medical model*, individuals are seen as responsible for neither problems nor solutions and are believed to need treatment. In the *enlightenment model*, actors are seen as responsible for problems but as unable or unwilling to provide solutions, and are believed to need discipline (Brickman et al., 1982, p.368). Few, if any, treatment centers ascribe to the moral model of helping and coping. In its logical extreme, no treatment is necessary since people's troubles are of their own making and exercising willpower is their solution (Fingarette, 1988). Programs that believe clients can only be cured by accepting the recovery regiment dictated by an external authority (charismatic leader or God) or spiritual community, and must confess the sinful behaviors of the past, subscribe to the enlightenment model of recovery. This includes most of the religious-based treatment centers, elements of the Alcoholics Anonymous community-based programs (Brickman,1982), and elements of most minority-based treatment programs. Since traditional treatment appears to have failed both African-American and Indian populations, synthesizing minorities' cultural heritage, spirituality, and religion with alcoholism treatment contains the best chances of recovery for ethnic groups (Rogan, 1986). This is most successfully administered by ethnic churches or spiritual leaders (Rogan, 1986; Slagle & Weibeo-Orlando, 1986). Therefore both religious and minority-based treatment centers primarily utilize elements of recovery that are associated with the enlightenment model of treatment.

Although adolescent treatment facilities vary somewhat in their approach to treatment, they seem to contain in common many elements found in the medical model approach (Silber, 1989; Zimmermen, 1990). Inherent in this model is the assumption that people are not responsible for the origin of or solution to their problems because they are subject to forces that are beyond their control, such as family circumstances. This assumption is manifested in a treatment structure that relies heavily on punitive behavior modification regiments (Darnton, 1989; Meacham, 1990; Allison et al., 1990; Schwartz, 1989) and family therapy (Kazdin et al., 1990; Szapocznik et al., 1990; Zimmerman, 1990).

In contrast, the majority of adult treatment programs contain elements of the compensatory model of helping and coping because they place more of an emphasis upon taking personal responsibility for recovery as found in Twelve Step program concepts (Bradley, 1988; Business Research Publications, 1991; Thurston et al., 1987). This results in a treatment structure that emphasizes psychoeducation, personal accountability, a more active participation in the recovery process, more control, self-reliance, a more egalitarian relationship between staff and patients, and abstinence supported by attending AA meetings (Alford et al., 1991; Francis, 1988; Gianetti, 1981; Business Research Publications, 1991; McCrady, 1990; Talbott, 1990). However some professionals argue that the AA-based treatment, with its reliance on using recovered alcoholics for therapists, who believe in a Higher Power, will foster the kind of dependency found in the medical model approach (Ellis & Schoenfeld, 1990).

For purposes of simplicity and while recognizing the enlightenment elements of submitting to a spiritual community (12 step meetings) for aftercare contained in both adolescent and adult models of helping, we will refer to the adolescent centers in terms of exemplifying the medical model, the adult centers, the compensatory model, and the religious/minority centers, the enlightenment model.

The enlightenment model of recovery, by nature, tends to look favorably upon treatment approaches that have an authority figure mandating a patient recovery regiment with strict behavior and moral guidelines. This leads to a paternalistic approach in treatment. Likewise, therapists tend to adopt this same authority role when treating adolescents only, thus acquiring a similar paternalistic attitude in the medical model of treatment (Silber, 1989). The major implications for treatment rendered is that therapists may assume that the knowlegeable medical professionals should usurp the right of the patient's decision-making (who is considered helpless), and, if neccessary, use coercive means to enforce the usurption (Silber, 1989). This eases the responsibility for recovery placed upon the adolescent and shifts it to an external source, such as the therapist or behavior control regiment (Darnton, 1989; Silber, 1989; Schwartz, 1989), family (French, 1987; Szapocznik et al., 1990), friends (Moorehouse, 1989), or environment (Needle et al., 1988). While recognizing that there are no pure models of treatment modalities, Brickman's classification scheme is most useful when the ascription of responsibility for a problem and its solution is important, as in the concept of paternalism (Silber, 1989).

The main research question addressed in this study is whether the focus on behavior management in adolescent-only treatment centers (Allison et al., 1989) has resulted in an increase in the counselors' paternalistic attitudes. We also wanted to know if this new focus in treatment has affected counselors' post-treatment abstinence expectations for adolescents. Finally, we were interested in discovering whether staff who are recovered chemical dependents would be more inclined than the staff who are not recovered to agree with a compensatory (as stressed by AA principles) rather than paternalistic approach.

We hypothesized that: (1) The religious and minority treatment center staff will report favoring more paternalistic treatment policies for all patient groups, followed by the adolescent-only treatment center staff, with the adult treatment center staff reporting the lowest level of paternalism. (2) The staff in adolescent-only treatment centers, when referring to a group of all-adolescent patient photographs, will prefer the more paternalistic solution to treatment problems than would the staff in the adult treatment centers. (3) All treatment center staff will predict lower rates of recovery for the adolescent patient appearing among pictures of all-adolescent patients than for the same adolescent picture appearing among pictures of all-adult patients. (4) Staff who are not recovered chemical dependents will be more paternalistic than staff who are recovered chemical dependents.

Method

Subjects

Subjects were 209 chemical dependency treatment staff who worked directly in a counseling capacity with patients. They were from thirty-one treatment clinics in seven USA states (AK, ID, NC, UT, VA, WA, WI). The thirty-one treatment clinics that participated in this study were selected from the telephone directory Yellow Pages based upon three criteria: their availability, proximity to the author's northern cross-country itinerary, and variety in type of treatment (adolescent-only, adult, minority and religious).

Materials

Materials consisted of a five page questionnaire with six pictures (3.5 X 5 cm) of either all adolescents or mostly adults followed by seven paternalistic versus compensatory treatment policy questions which concerned controls on music, dress codes, swearing, canteen priviledges, the emphasis placed on family therapy, and taking personal responsibility for avoiding relapse, four of which were Likert-type questions ranging from "strongly disagree" (1) to "strongly agree" (5) and three of which were forced two-choice responses, two write-in response questions, one asking about the chances of Phil's recovery, an adolescent whose picture appeared in both groups of pictures (all-adolescent and mostly-adult) and the other asking how many AA meetings per month the therapist recommended, along with eight demographic questions. In order to establish the validity of the questionnaire, five judges read the definitions of paternalistic and compensatory approaches to addiction treatment and classified the questionnaire choices into each approach. All judges' responses were consistent on all items except for two, which had an 80 percent agreement rate.

Procedure

The clinic director was contacted personally to obtain permission to administer the questionnaire. The directors and individual staff were told that the purpose of the study was to contribute knowledge about the adolescent recovery process by measuring staff treatment attitudes. The director was asked to hand the questionnaires to all counseling staff members with instructions that participation was voluntary and anonymous. Half the staff randomly received one picture configuration (six adolescents), while the other half received the other (one adolescent and five adults).

Results

Treatment Centers

Thirty-one of the forty-one treatment clinics approached participated in the study (see Table 1 for selected parameters), yielding an institutional response rate of 75.6 percent. The staff's responses to the seven policy questions were summed to yield a paternalistic scale score. This value was used to compare the degree of paternalism in treatment approaches among the three types of clinics, adolescent-only, adult, and religious/minority. A oneway ANOVA revealed there was a significant difference in paternalism among types of treatment programs (F (2,192) = 6.88, p < .002). A multiple comparison follow-up, using Sheffe's procedure, found that the religious and minority treatment centers were significantly more paternalistic than the adolescent-only and adult treatment centers, partially confirming the first hypothesis. The adolescent-only and adult treatment clinics' scores were not significantly different (see Table 2).

Table 1.

Selected Parameters for Particpating Programs

Program	State	Type	Year Open	Days Open	Hrs	Environments Served	Population Served	Fees	Techniques Used	Max # Clients	# Staff	Staff/Patient Ratio
1	WA	bcdh	1971	7	24	abce	i	a	aef	n.r.	n.r.	1:8
2	WA	ab	n.r.	7	24	bc	ad	bcg	abcdh	36	18	1:5
3	WA	abe	1978	7	24	abc	ah	bcd	ab	34	51	1:5
4	WA	bg	1984	7	24	abce	a	bg	abd	72	20	n.r.
5	WA	fg	1976	7	24	e	j	f	aij	255	10	n.r.
6	WA	ab	1988	7	24	abc	di	bcg	abcde	17	28	1:4
7	WA	ab	1988	7	24	abc	aki	bcde	abce	24	28	1:4
8	WA	b	1985	5	12	abc	ad	bcf	abce	250	8	n.r.
9	WA	abe	1982	7	24	abc	ad	bcd	abcdg	162	40	1:7
10	NC	g	1958	7	24	bc	bk	f	bdi	30	4	1:10
11	NC	g	1983	7	24	bc	b	a	abcd	9	6	1:8
12	NC	g	1977	7	24	abce	e	bf	bij	20	12	1:5
13	NC	a	1971	7	24	abc	a	dc	abcd	48	67	1:2
14	NC	g	1989	7	24	abc	d	bdg	abce	28	19	1:10
15	WI	b	1986	5	9	e	jk	f	abf	75	4	1:10
16	WI	ac	1982	7	24	ab	ad	cf	a	20	20	1:2.5
17	WI	ah	1983	7	24	abce	a	a	ab	30	50	1:5
18	WI	abe	1988	7	24	abc	ad	bcd	abcd	17	26	1:2
19	WI	g	1989	7	24	c	j	g	abd	8	4	1:2
20	ID	g	1987	7	24	abc	f	bc	abdg	20	22	1:1
21	ID	i	1970	n.a.	n.a.	bc	a	g	adk	n.r.	3	n.r.
22	ID	ab	1986	7	24	bc	adg	ac	ace	15	18	1:3
23	ID	a	1986	5	9	c	d	ac	ace	250	12	n.r.
24	ID	b	1988	5	11	bcd	d	abc	acl	n.r.	3	n.r.
25	UT	ab	n.r.	7	24	ab	ad	bcd	abcd	n.r.	n.r.	n.r.
26	UT	g	1954	7	24	e	b	a	dm	60	12	1:5
27	UT	g	1977	7	24	abcde	d	bgh	abceg	23	17	1:3
28	AK	abc	1985	7	24	abcd	dg	bcdg	abm	40	n.r.	1:5
29	AK	fd	1977	5	9	ab	d	f	abhi	150	30	1:4.5
30	AK	g	1989	7	24	cd	k	g	n	15	4	1:3
31	VA	ab	1988	7	24	abc	d	bcdg	abd	32	40	1:2.5

Key to Table 1.

Type of program

a=In-patient	d=Emergency response	g=Residential
b=Out-patient	e=Day treatment services	h=Community intervention
c=Detoxification	f=Storefront ministry	i=Parole

Environments served

a=Urban	c=Rura	e=Inner city
b=Suburban	d=Reservation/Tribe	

Populations served

a=Adults	e=Male adolescents only	i=Pregnant
b=Men only	f=Female adolescents only	j=Indigent/low income
c=Women only	g=Children	k=Minority
d=Adolescents	h=Elderly	

Fees

a=Government subsidy (sliding scale)	d=Medicaid	g=Government subsidy (fixed fee)
b=Private payment	e=Medicare	h=Tribal funds
	f=No fee/donations	

c=Insurance
Treatment Techniques Used

a=Individual counseling	f=Crisis counseling	k=Punitive
b=Group therapy	g=Outdoor challenges	l=Peer support
c=Education/lectures	h=Recreational	m=Cognitive
d=Family therapy	i=Biblical ministry	n=Cultural
e=Twelve Step/AA/NA	j=Work	

Note: n.r.=no response   n.a.=not applicable.

Table 2.
Mean Staff Demographic Values for Adolescent, Adult, and Religious/ Minority Treatment Center Models

| | | Model | |
Characteristic	Adolescent	Adult	Religious/Minority
Age			
M	36.5	42.1	40.0
SD	9.1	9.0	9.7
Range	19-63	22-56	24-68
Years in field			
M	5.1	6.2	4.9
SD	4.0	4.9	4.8
Range	0-21	0-19	.2-18
Yrs. advanced education			
M	3.4	3.0	1.8
SD	2.1	2.4	2.1
Range	0-9	0-9	0-6
Paternalism score			
M	12.8	13.1	15.2
SD	2.8	2.9	3.2
Range	8-19	6-19	9-21
Religiousness	2.8	2.4	3.0
% Female	60.3	57.9	50.0
% Minority	14.2	8.8	8.8/100
% Recovered alcoholic	22.8	54.2	52.0

Note: Religiousness (which includes Twelve Step program activities) is coded 1=low (0-2 religious activities/yr.); 2=medium (1-2 religious activities/mo.); 3=high (1-2 religious activities/wk.).

The adolescent-only treatment center staff responded significantly more paternalistically overall (t (50) = 2.51; p < .01) to the adolescent patient photographs (M = 13.68; N = 28), as predicted in the second hypothesis, than the adult patient photographs (M = 11.79; N = 24), while the adult and religious/minority staff groups did not significantly differ on either set.

Staff

The third hypothesis was not supported. There was no significant difference in the staff's predictions about the chances of patients' recovery between the adolescent and adult photo groups. However, most therapists reported unrealistic chances of recovery for their patients. Only 17.7 percent expected abstinence chances to be 15 percent or less, 32.3 percent expected abstience chances to lie between 15 and 30 percent, and 50 percent expected abstinence chances to be 30 percent or greater ($\underline{M}$ = 36.9%; $\underline{SD}$ = 21.0).

In partial support of the fourth hypothesis, recovered alcoholic/addicts responded in a less paternalistic manner than the non-alcoholic staff to three treatment characteristic questions: family therapy ($\underline{t}$ (192) = 2.23; p < .02) ($\underline{M}$ = 3.09; $\underline{N}$ = 88 vs $\underline{M}$ = 3.72; $\underline{N}$ = 106); relapse ($\underline{t}$ (192) = 2.02; p < .03) ($\underline{M}$ = 3.16; $\underline{N}$ = 87 vs. $\underline{M}$ = 3.73, $\underline{N}$ = 107); and personal responsibility in recovery for avoiding chemical using friends ($\underline{t}$ (196) = 3.05; p < .002; $\underline{M}$ = 1.67, $\underline{N}$ = 90 vs. $\underline{M}$ = 2.41, $\underline{N}$ = 108).

With regard to all staff, their relative degree of reported paternalism was highest in the treatment characteristics of music, dress, family therapy and relapse. They responded with more compensatory policies on the characteristics of swearing and making lifestyle changes, which is broken down by treatment modality in Table 3.

Table 3.

Mean Paternalism Scores as a Function of Treatment Model

Characteristic	N	Model		
		Adult	Adolescent	Religious/minority
Music control	209			
M		3.63	3.48	4.38
SD		1.48	1.43	.86
Swearing control	208			
M		2.47	2.72	3.38
SD		1.46	1.40	1.61
Canteen Control	208			
M		2.45	2.19	3.00
SD		1.38	1.33	1.46
Dress codes	208			
M		3.57	3.53	3.28
SD		1.44	1.26	1.51
Family therapy	201			
M		3.50	3.67	2.66
SD		1.94	1.90	2.01
Relapse	201			
M		3.20	3.85	4.17
SD		2.00	1.83	1.65
Lifestyle changes	205			
M		2.21	1.91	1.83
SD		1.85	1.69	1.65

Note: The scores ranged from 1 to 5, with 5 denoting a high degree of paternalism in the therapists' approach to treatment.

A Posteriori Analyses

The recovered alcoholics were disproportionately represented in the adult treatment centers (_(1, N = 78) = 15.42; p < .001), where 54 percent of all staff (N = 65) were recovered alcoholics versus 23 percent (N = 13) in adolescent-only treatment centers. Recovered alcoholic/addict counselors recommended significantly more AA meetings (t (171) = 3.49; p < .001) for clients (M = 16.87 meetings per month) than non-alcoholic counselors (M = 11.87 meetings per month).

Both adolescent and adult treatment center staff recommended more AA meetings per month for adults than adolescents (F (1,175) = 5.06; p < .03), with the religious/minority center staff recommending only half as many AA meetings than the adult center staff for adults (t (19) = 2.90, p < .01) as shown in Table 4.

Table 4.
Mean Number of AA Meetings Recommended per Month as a Function of the Type of Treatment Model and Picture Grouping

Treatment Model	Picture grouping	
	All-adolescent	Mostly-Adult
Adolescent	12.41	14.31
Adult	14.33	18.21
Religious/minority	11.20	9.46

Discussion

Results support part of the first hypothesis, that religious/minority centers were significantly more paternalistic in their policies to all patients than adult or adolescent-only models. Contrary to the rest of the hypothesis, the adult and adolescent-only centers did not differ significantly from each other on the overall paternalism scale, possibly because the staff from adult treatment centers were more paternalistic than their presumed philosophies would suggest. We found, as hypothesized, that staff in adolescent-only centers generally treat adolescent patients in a more paternalistic manner than adult patients, while the staff in adult centers do not treat adolescents and adults differently. Also contrary to our predictions, all treatment center staff did not predict lower rates of recovery for the adolescent, Phil, when seen with all adolescent cohorts than with adult fellow patients. Staff recovery predictions were so erratic, ranging from 0 to 100 percent in all centers, it appears they are not well informed about the research findings on treatment outcome. Finally, we had partial confirmation of the hypothesis that recovered chemical dependent staff would be less paternalistic than the non-dependent staff.

The major limitations of this study are that an available, rather than random, sample of treatment centers was used, which opens the possibility of sampling bias. Also, the stimuli were pictures, rather than real patients, possibly posing generalizability problems from pictures to real patients. In addition, there is no universally agreed upon definition of paternalism. These limitations should be kept in mind when interpreting the results of this study.

The adult treatment therapists' scores were surprisingly high on the paternalistic side of the scale, more in line with the medical model of treatment ("Do as I say"), than compensatory ("How can I help you") even though most adult centers are described as basically compensatory in their approach (Francis, 1988; Gianetti, 1981; Business Research Publications, 1991; McCrady, 1990; Talbott, 1990). At first glance, this finding would seem to support the contention of Ellis & Schoenfeld (1990), that AA-based treatment undermines the compensatory philosophy of "self-reliance and self-control." However, when testing the recovered alcoholics separately for paternalistic policies, their paternalism score decreased on three treatment interventions, in partial confirmation of our fourth hypothesis. In other words, a recovering alcoholic is more likely to be compensatory than his/her fellow staff members, supporting the counterarguments that AA concepts mean an assumption of patient personal accountability, self-control and self-reliance.

Two of the current findings indicate adolescent-only treatment center staff may view addiction differently than adult treatment center staff. Although it is generally considered good therapy for recovering chemical dependents to relate to others in recovery, and therefore be on the staff of recovery centers (Bradley, 1988; Ellis & Schoenfeld, 1990), there are relatively few chemical dependent recovered staff represented on the adolescent-only units. Bradley (1988), in her review of AA and treatment, stated that up to 60 percent of staff in all treatment centers were recovering from alcoholism themselves. We found this not to be true in adolescent centers, where only 23 percent of the staff were recovered addict/alcoholics, but confirmed her conclusion in the adult centers by finding that 54 percent of staff there were recovered alcoholic/addicts.

Also it is well documented that AA (Twelve Step) meetings during and after treatment increase significantly the chances of abstinence following treatment (Alford et al., 1991; Bradley, 1988; Brown et al., 1989; Thurstin et al., 1987; Vaillant & Milofsky, 1982), but we found that adolescent-only center staff recommend fewer meetings per month for adolescents than adult center patients. This may indicate that the goals in adolescent treatment centers may not be consistent with adult treatment.

In sum, these findings suggest a number of implications for chemical dependency counselors. All types of chemical dependency counselors need to become more knowledgable about what the research evidence indicates are the abstinence chances of their patients. The religious/minority counselors should be aware that they are not emphasizing the use of Twelve Step programs as much as the regular adult program counselors, which would indicate they are not aware of the research on the effectiveness of Twelve Step program aftercare for abstinence. The greater degree of paternalism favored in treatment by religious/minority counselors for all patients, and adolescent counselors for adolescents, than that preferred by regular adult treatment counselors, indicates the efficacy of the paternalistic versus compensatory approach for different chemical dependent populations needs to be examined in future research studies.

References

Alford, G. S., Koehler, R. A. & Leonard, J. Alcoholics Anonymous-Narcotics Anonymous model in-patient treatment of chemically dependent adolescents: A two year outcome study. *J. Stud. Alco.* 52: 118-126, 1991.

Allison, K., Leone, P. E. & Spero, E. R. Drug and alcohol use among adolescents: Social context and competence. In: Leone, P. (Ed.), *Understanding Troubled and Troubling Youth*, pp. 173-193, Newberry Park, CA: Sage Publications, 1990.

Bradley, A. M. Keep coming back. *Alco. Health Resear. World.* 12: 193-199, 1988.

Brickman, P., Rabinowitz, C., Daruza, J., Coates, D., Cohn, E. & Kidder, L. Models of helping and coping. *Amer. Psychol.* 37: 368-384, 1982.

Brown, S. A. Vik, P. W. & Creamer, V. A. Characteristics of relapse following adolescent substance abuse treatment. *Addic. Behav.*, 14: 291-300, 1989.

Business Research Publications. Bringing humane care to treating alcohol and drug abuse. *Subs. Abuse Report.* Vol XX, No 11 (ISSN 1040-4164) p 6-7. 1991.

Darnton, N. Committed youth. *Newsweek.* July, 66-72, 1989.

Ellis, A. & Schoenfeld, E. Divine Intervention and the treatment of chemical dependency. *J. Subs. Abuse.* 2: 459-468, 1990.

Fingarette, H. Alcoholism: The mythical disease. *Pub. Inter.*, 91: 3-33, 1988.

Francis, R. J. Update on alcohol and drug disorder treatment. *J. Clin. Psychi.*, 49: 13-17, 1988.

French, S. Family approaches to alcoholism; Why the lack of interest among marriage and family professionals? *J . Drug Iss.*, 17, 359-368, 1987.

Friedman, A. S., Glickman, N. W. & Morrissey, M. R. Prediction to successful treatment outcome by client characteristics and retention in treatment in adolescent drug treatment programs: a large-scale cross validation study. *J. Drug Educ.* 16: 149-165, 1986.

Gianetti, V. Alcoholics Anonymous and the recovering alcoholic: An exploratory study. *Amer. J. Drug Alco. Abuse.* 8: 363-370, 1981.

Kazdin, A. E., Ayers, W. A., Bass, D. & Rodgers, A. Empirical and clinical focus of child and adolescent psychotherapy research. *J. Consul. Clin. Psycho.* 58: 729-740, 1990.

Marlatt, G. A., Baer, J. S., Donovan, D. M. & Kivlahan, D. R. Addictive behaviors: etiology and treatment. In: Rosenzweig, M. R. & Porter, L. W. (Eds.) *Annual Review of Psychology*, 39: 223-252, Annual Reviews Inc., Palo Alto, CA, 1988.

McCrady, B. The divine, the saturnine and the internecine: comments on Ellis and Schoenfeld. *J. of Subs. Abuse*, 2:477-480, 1990.

Meacham, A. Adolescent treatment programs come of age. *U.S. J. Drug Alco. Depen.* 13: 1, 5, 1989.

Meacham, A. Abuses tarnish adolescent treatment. *U.S. J. Drug Alco. Depen.* 14: 1,7. 1990.

Morehouse, E. R. Treating adolescent alcohol abusers. Social Casework: *J. Contem. Social Work*, June: 355-363, 1989.

Needle, R., Su, S., Doherty, W., Lavee, Y. & Brown, P. Familial, interpersonal, and intrapersonal correlates of drug use: A longitudinal comparison of adolescents in treatment, drug using adolescents not in treatment and non-drug using adolescents. *Inter. J. Addic.*, 23: 1211-1240, 1988.

Piercy, F. P. & Frankel, B. R. The evolution of an integrative family therapy for substance abusing abolescents: Toward the mutual enhancement of research and practice. *J. Fam. Psycho.* 3: 5-25, 1989.

Reichelt, S. & Christensen B. Reflections during a study on family therapy with drug addicts. *Fam. Proc.* 29: 273-287, 1990.

Rogan, A. Recovery from alcoholism issues for Black and Native American alcoholics. *Alco. Health and Resear. World.* 11: 42-44, 1986.

Schwartz, I. *(In)Justice for Juveniles: Rethinking the Best Interests of the Child.* Lexington, MA: Lexington Books, 1989.

Silber, T. J. Justified paternalism in adolescent health care. *J. Adol. Health Care,* 10: 449-453. 1989.

Slagle, A. L. & Weibel-Orlando, J. The Indian Shaker Church and Alcoholics Anonymous: Revitalistic curing cults. *Human Organi.* 45: 310-317, 1986.

Szapocznik, J., Kurtines, W., Santisteban, D. A. & Rio, A. T. Interplay of advances between theory, research and application in treatment interventions aimed at behavior problem children and adolescents. *J. Consul. Clin. Psycho.* 58: 696-703, 1990.

Taffaro, C. & Forsyth, C. J. The effect of living arrangement on the recovery of adolescent alcoholics: A research note. *Free Inquir. Creative Sociol.,* 17: 163-164, 1989.

Talbott, G. D. Commentary on "Divine intervention and the treatment of chemical dependency." *J. Subs. Abuse,* 2: 469-471. 1990.

Thurstin, A. H., Alfano, A. M. & Nerviano, V. T. The efficacy of AA attendance for aftercare of in-patient alcoholics: Some follow-up data. *Int. J. Addic.* 22: 1083-1090, 1987.

Vaillant, G. & Milofsky, E. Natural history of male alcoholism. IV. Paths to recovery. *Arch. Gen. Psychi.* 39: 127-133, 1982.

Zimmermen, P. Notes on the history of adolescent in-patient and residential treatment. *Adoles.* 25: 12-38, 1990.

Appendix 2

Adolescent Recovery Rate

The figure of "less than 5 percent recovery rate," is a calculated estimate. It was derived using: observation, experience, and the preliminary results of a new study now being conducted.

Numerous treatment programs were observed on a nation-wide research tour of seventy-five treatment centers for chemically dependent youth. Treatment center personnel most frequently asked the question, "How high is the recovery rate in other centers?" The answer was "very poor." The response to this was one of relief because these centers' results were also poor. There was also concern that the odds were not improving.

A 98 percent failure rate was experienced by most of these centers according to the personnel who anonymously provided this information.

Even though most brochures for treatment centers cite a 75 to 80 percent success rate, it is believed these are inflated statistics. Either the statistics are based on how many kids *leave* treatment clean and sober, telephone self-report follow-ups are used, or "success" is defined as getting along better at home and in school. These methods of collecting data do not give reliable information: leaving treatment is not recovery. when leaving treatment is not recovery. In addition, denial and lying are hallmarks of the disease of addiction, thus making the "self-report" statistics useless. And if getting along at home is the goal—why are they in an addiction treatment center?

Although some adolescents remained clean and sober after treatment (showing me enough successful components of treatment to justify this book), they almost always said they were the *only* one of their fellow patients who made it. The most careful research reviews reveal that less than 15 percent of people remain abstinent post-treatment (1). We also know adolescent abstinence is less than adults (2).

Treatment can work. Many of the adolescents who went through treatment in the young people's program developed at St. Luke's Hospital are still clean and sober. Many of the young alcoholics that worked on *Young, Sober, & Free* in 1978 are also clean and sober.

But when I put my daughter into treatment, *not one single patient remained clean and sober coming out of treatment*. This included about twenty adolescents in a forty-five day program. That meant a 100 percent failure rate. In addition, in aftercare, no sober former patients could be found to support their on-going group. It was dismal, but not uncommon.

In the research for this book, 225 questionnaires were sent to seventy-five adolescent treatment facilities. These were to be filled out by patients and treatment graduates with either thirty days, nine months or one year of sobriety. Of the questionnaires returned only one treatment center located a graduate sober for a full year. Although successes of treatment do not hang around hospital units, sober people from treatment generally remain available in some form.

Combined with my experience, this survey indicates the conclusion that more questionnaires with adolescents maintaining a year of sobriety were not returned because they could not be found. There are not many.

For these reasons, stated 5 percent success rate may be too generous. I am currently engaged in on-going research headed by Dr. Michael Marshall, research psychologist. It consists of surveying young people who attempted to get clean and sober in their teenage years. Because it has proved so difficult to track patients from treatment through recovery, we are trying a novel approach—studying the clean and sober adolescent *back* through treatment. In other words, what finally works in adolescent recovery.

Preliminary results show overwhelmingly that adolescents who enter standard adult treatment are four to five times more likely to find sobriety than adolescents who go through adolescent-only units. The pilot study, "Homogeneous versus Heterogeneous Age Group Treatment of Adolescent Substance Abusers" was published in the *American Journal of Alcohol and Drug Abuse* (see Appendix 3).

Endnotes

1. Marlatt, G. A., Baer, J.S., Donovan, D.M. & Kivlahan, D. R. Addictive behaviors: etiology and treatment. In: Rosenzweig, M.R. & Porter, L.W. (Eds.) *Annual Review of Psychology*, 39: 223-252, Annual Reviews Inc., Palo Alto, CA, 1988.

2. Filatead, W. J. (Director of Study). Two-year treatment outcome. Parkside Medical Services Corporation, 205 West Touchy Ave., Park Ridge, Illinois 60068.

Appendix 3

Homogeneous Versus Heterogeneous Age Group Treatment of Adolescent Substance Abusers

Michael J. Marshall, Ph.D., North Carolina A & T State University
Shelly Marshall, BS, Youth Enjoying Sobriety Retreat
Correspondence should be addressed to: Michael J. Marshall, Ph.D., Department of Psychology, North Carolina A & T State University, Greensboro, NC 27411

Abstract

The treatment outcome from homogeneous age group substance abuse treatment centers, whose clientele consisted primarily of adolescent substance abusers, was compared to heterogeneous age group substance abuse treatment centers, where adolescent and adult patients were treated together. Subjects were 100 substance abusers, from twenty states, who recovered in adolescence and had at least eleven months of continuous abstinence. A twenty-four item self-report questionnaire was used to ascertain the type of recovery treatment experienced, number of relapses, and duration of sobriety. Results indicated a disproportionate number of substance abusers who recovered in adolescence were treated in a heterogeneous age group clinical setting. There was no significant difference in the length of sobriety and number of relapses between the homogeneous and heterogeneous treatment groups. These data suggest adolescent substance abusers can be treated at a lower cost and with a higher recovery rate by placing them in adult treatment settings.

Homogeneous Versus Heterogeneous Age Group Treatment Of Adolescent Substance Abusers

Approximately 115,000 adolescents are treated each year in the United States for substance abuse (1). One of the decisions that must be made before treatment can begin is whether to place an adolescent substance abuser in a homogeneous age group treatment environment, where all patients are adolescents, or a heterogeneous age group treatment environment, where adults and adolescents are treated together (2, 3, 4, 5).

Most adolescent substance abusers are placed in a homogeneous treatment center (1) because it is assumed to have a positive impact on the treatment outcome. The rationale for this assumption rests upon the belief that homogeneous age grouping offers certain benefits over heterogeneous age grouping (3, 4). Peer grouping has been claimed to reduce feelings of isolation, increase the motivation to abstain through peer support, and allow the staff to tailor treatment to meet unique adolescent needs (2, 3, 6).

However, this assumption can be questioned on the grounds that certain negative aspects of homogeneous age grouping may offset the benefits. For instance, adolescents in trouble have a tendency, when grouped together, to create negative bonding which is manifested in a number of ways. It can create an us-against-them mentality, and lead to the mutual reinforcement of bad habits and the desire to resist authority (7, 8, 9). The staff can actually elicit problem behaviors through self-fulfilling prophecies if they expect teenagers to act up when together (10, 11). In addition, the excessive reliance on rules and regulations to govern behavior in a youth treatment structure can lead to a feeling of deprivation on the part of the adolescent living in such a highly restrictive environment (9, 12, 13). And finally, homogeneous age grouping precludes the benefits that can be conferred by the presence of mature role models (14).

While the case for the superiority of heterogeneous age grouping has not as yet been empirically tested in a substance abuse treatment setting, research from other disciplines suggests the idea may have some merit. The issue of homogeneous versus heterogeneous ability grouping has been researched extensively in the field of education. Tracking in education has been found to have several negative repercussions on those who are placed in homogeneous ability groups (11). Slavin (15), in a review of the ability grouping literature, cites a number of arguments against ability grouping. Those in the lower achievement groups are deprived of high achieving role models, underachieve due to fulfilling low expectations, exhibit low self-esteem, and are more disruptive than those in heterogeneous groups. Slavin concludes that all students would benefit most from identifying primarily with a heterogeneous classroom group. Overall, the research results to date indicate that students achieve more when heterogeneously grouped. This has led to a national "effective schools" movement, termed cooperative learning, where students of mixed ability are put together because they help each other learn better.

In a conceptually related study, Radziszewska and Rogoff (16) examined the effect of heterogeneous age grouping directly in a learning task. They studied the influence of peer versus adult collaboration on ten year olds' ability to learn errand planning skills and found the children's performance to be superior in the heterogeneous age groups due to the benefits resulting from adult guidance.

In light of these findings from education demonstrating the superiority of heterogeneous grouping on achievement, the presumed superiority of homogeneous age grouping in adolescents' substance abuse treatment should not remain an untested assumption. Due to the difficulty of keeping track of adolescents from treatment in follow-up studies (17, 18, 19), this research question was examined in this study with an after-the-fact approach to identifying successful treatment variables. Recovered adolescent substance abusers were found by approaching places where sober youth congregate. Those who had remained abstinent for at least 11 months were asked about the type of treatment they experienced. The assumption was that the most successful treatment modality (homogeneous verses heterogeneous age grouping) could be identified by the presence of a disproportionate number of representatives. Two dependent variables were measured, the number of relapses since treatment, and the duration of total abstinence. It was hypothesized that those who were treated as adolescents in heterogeneous age group settings would be disproportionately represented among those with eleven or more months sobriety, would have a longer duration of total abstinence, and would have fewer relapses than those treated in homogeneous age group settings.

Method

Subjects

The subjects were 205 available recovered substance abusers who first attempted sobriety in adolescence and had at least eleven months of continuous sobriety at the time they participated in this study. Originally twelve months of abstinence was chosen as the measure of treatment response because it is a commonly accepted criterion for treatment success (20,21,22). However, three subjects, who reported being close to a year of abstinence (eleven mos.), were not discarded from the analysis because there is evidence it would not change statistically the outcome of treatment (23). Their place of residence spanned twenty states. Subjects volunteered to participate in the study in exchange for a bumper sticker. Data from sixty-four subjects was not analyzed because they improperly filled out the questionnaire or did not meet the abstinence duration requirements. Forty-one subjects attained abstinence without clinical treatment, leaving 100 subjects in the study. Their ages ranged from fifteen through thirty-eight years, 9 percent were minorities (four Hispanic, three African-American, and two Native-American), and there were fifty-five males and forty-five females.

Materials

A self-report twenty-four item questionnaire that measured substance abuse, treatment, demographic variables, and relapse and abstinence history was used. Sample questions were: *What was your primary drug of choice? What type of treatment were you taken to the first time? (please check one): Adolescent chemical dependency hospital unit; Adolescent treatment-not hospital; Adolescent religious center; Adult chemical dependency hospital unit; Adult treatment-not hospital; Adult religious center; Other. Have you been clean and sober continuously since your first attempt at sobriety? If you have not been clean and sober continuously since your first attempt at sobriety, how many times have you relapsed?*

Procedure

Potential subjects were approached throughout the United States from February through November of 1990 in places where teenage and adult recovered substance abusers were likely to congregate, such as the 1990 AA World Convention, Alcoholics Anonymous, Narcotics Anonymous, and Cocaines Anonymous meetings, twelve step clubs, treatment center follow-up programs, Campus Crusade for Christ, high school drug programs and Indian reservation treatment programs. Forty percent of the questionnaires were administered by the second author and two volunteers at the 1990 AA World Convention in the Young People's Hospitality Suite, 38 percent were administered by the second author at various locations with proximity to her northern cross-country itinerary, and the remainder (22 percent) were administered by volunteers in Salt Lake City (UT), Beloit, Whitewater, and Milwaukee (WI), and Anchorage (AK).

Respondents were handed a questionnaire individually and given these instructions, "This is a questionnaire investigating how teenage substance abusers recover. It is voluntary and anonymous. It takes about 10 minutes to finish. In exchange for your time, you can have a free *Day By Day* or *Young, Sober, & Free* bumper sticker, whether or not you choose to fill out the questionnaire. I will answer any questions you may have while filling out the questionnaire." Respondents were thanked upon turning in the questionnaire and given a bumper sticker.

Results

The proportion of respondents reporting a heterogeneous or homogeneous treatment environment was calculated. Of those who underwent clinical treatment, 59 percent (n=59) were treated in a homogeneous age group facility and 41 percent (n=41) were treated in a heterogeneous age group facility. This proportion represents the relative success of each treatment type (homogeneous verses heterogeneous). The proportion of adolescents actually admitted to heterogeneous or homogeneous age clinical settings is reported to be 84.5 percent homogeneous and 16.5 percent heterogeneous (1). A test for the significance of a proportion (24) revealed adolescents recovered in a significantly greater than expected proportion from the heterogeneous age group programs ($z = 7.53$, $p < .001$), as hypothesized. In order to determine whether this finding interacts with gender, a separate test for the significance of a proportion was calculated for males and females. Both genders were significantly overrepresented in the heterogeneous treatment setting. Sixty-nine and one tenth percent of the males (n=38) were treated in a homogeneous setting verses 30.9 percent (n=17) treated in a heterogeneous setting ($z = 3.16$, $p < .001$). Forty six and seven tenths percent of the females (n=21) were treated in a homogeneous setting verses 53.3 percent (n=24) treated in a heterogeneous setting ($z = 7.01$, $p < .001$). Contrary to the remaining hypotheses, no significant difference was found in the length of total abstinence nor the relapse rate between the two types of treatment settings. The standard significance level of $\propto = .05$ was used in this study.

An independent means t-test showed the mean age of first attempted sobriety is significantly older ($t(98) = 3.45$; $p < .01$) for those adolescents treated in a heterogeneous setting ($M = 16.8$, $SD = 2.3$) than for those treated in a homogeneous setting ($M = 15.5$, $SD = 1.5$). A chi-square analysis revealed that males and females differentially appear in

Homogeneous vs. Heterogeneous Age Group Treatment
of Adolescent Substance Abusers

treatment settings, with significantly more males treated in homogeneous settings and significantly more females treated in heterogeneous settings $(\chi^2(1) = 5.14,\ p < .05)$

Table 1.
Selected Characteristics of Recovered Substance Abusers Who Were Treated in Adolescence for Homogeneous and Heterogeneous Settings

Characteristic	Homogeneous (n=59)		Heterogeneous (n=41)	
	N	%	N	%
Pretreatment				
Sex				
Male	38	64.4	17	41.5
Female	21	35.6	24	58.5
Primary Drug of Choice				
Alcohol	27	45.8	17	41.5
Marijuana	13	22.0	13	31.7
Crack/cocaine	9	15.3	5	12.2
Amphetamines	3	5.1	3	7.3
LSD/PCP	5	8.5	1	2.4
Barbiturates	1	1.7	1	2.4
Heroin	1	1.7	1	2.4
Treatment				
Type of Program				
Hospital unit	29	49.2	23	56.1
Non-hospital (clinic or residential)	29	49.2	17	41.5
Religious center	1	1.7	1	2.4
Post-Treatment				
Number of Post-treatment Relapses				
No Relapse	27	47.4	19	47.5
Minor Relapse (1-3)	18	31.6	12	30.0
Major Relapse (4 or more)	14	21.0	10	22.5
	Mean	SD	Mean	SD
Number of Years Elapsed				
Since Treatment	4.1	2.7	6.4	4.6
Years Abstinent	3.0	2.1	3.8	3.8

Discussion

The finding that there is a disproportionate number of recovered substance abusers who were treated in adolescence from heterogeneous age group clinical settings than from homogeneous age group clinical settings supports the hypothesis that a heterogeneous setting offers a higher probability of recovery for adolescent substance abusers. However, the lack of any differences in length of sobriety or number of relapses suggests the quality of sobriety, for those who do recover, does not differ between the two settings.

The validity of self-report data, such as those reported in this study, is questionable to some (25). However, in a review of the literature, Hesselbrock et al. (26) concluded post-hospitalization self-reports of drinking behavior were highly correlated with reports provided by official records, documents and collateral informants. Furthermore, in the present study, the validity of self-reports of abstinence are increased by the fact that the subjects were exhibiting an abstinent lifestyle, characterized by attending the aftercare programs where these data were collected.

Another question relating to the validity of these findings concerns selection bias. Were those addicts who recovered in heterogeneous settings more likely to be present at the data collection locations? It does not seem likely due to their wide geographical range (twenty states) and the wide variety of settings visited (from the AA World Convention to Indian reservation treatment programs). In addition, research has shown that the majority of all recovered substance abusers rely upon twelve step programs to maintain their sobriety (27, 28), where most subjects in this study were obtained.

A potentially more troubling issue concerns the confounds that are always present in correlational research. The finding that adolescents treated in heterogeneous settings were about sixteen months older could challenge the notion that a heterogeneous setting is superior, that is, if sixteen year old adolescents are more likely to benefit from treatment than fifteen year old adolescents. Another confound concerns whether outcome differences resulted from different social dynamics in heterogeneous settings or different treatment techniques. Correlational findings cannot be used to distinguish which is the case, but they are still valuable in that they can point to promising areas of future research that can be designed to reveal which specific variables are critical in leading to superior outcomes.

The implications of these findings are significant for treatment because many professionals and insurers are demanding cost justification and outcome accountability in adolescent substance abuse treatment (29, 4). Since units serving higher proportions of young clients have a significantly higher staffing ratio (199 to 271 paid staff per 1000 clients compared to all units at 140 paid staff per 1000 clients) [1] and spend about two weeks longer in treatment (29), units serving a high proportion of young clients cost more. This higher cost is probably a reflection of the additional youth specific interventions provided by adolescent treatment centers. If, as these data suggest, youth are less likely to recover when placed in youth treatment, then placing adolescents in the adult treatment centers would not only be more cost effective, but would also increase recovery rates. In conclusion, these initial findings, although correlational in nature, suggest the heterogeneous age grouping superiority effect may warrant further research attention.

References

(1) National Institute of Drug Abuse and National Institute on Alcohol Abuse and Alcoholism. (1990). Summary of NDATUS findings on youth. *1989 National Drug and Alcoholism Treatment Unit Survey* (DHHS Publication No. ADM 89-1630). Washington, DC: U. S. Government Printing Office.

(2) Meacham, A. (1989). Adolescent treatment programs come of age. U.S. *J. Drug Alcohol Depen.*, *13*, 1, 5.

(3) Morehouse, E. R. (1989). Treating adolescent alcohol abusers. *Social Case Work: J. Contem. Social Work*, June, 355-363.

(4) Newcomb, M. D., & Bentler P. M. (1989). Substance use and abuse among children and teenagers. *Am. Psychol.*, *44*, 242-248A.

(5) Morrison, M. A. (1990). Addiction in adolescents. *Wes. J. Med.*, *152*, 543-546.

(6) Unger R. A. (1978). The treatment of adolescent alcoholism. *Social Casework*, *59*, 27-35.

(7) Donovan, J. E., & Jessor, R. (1985). Structure of problem behavior in adolescence and young adulthood. *J. Consult. Clin. Psychol.*, *53*, 890-904.

(8) Tannehill, R. L. (1987). Employing a modified positive peer culture treatment approach in a state youth center. *J. Offen. Counsel. Serv. Rehab.*, *12*, 113-129

(9) Fraiser, G., & Sullivan D. (1989). *Burnt*. New York: NAC Books.

(10) Rosenbaum, J. E. (1980). Social implications of educational grouping. *Rev. Resear. Educ.*, *8*, 361-401.

(11) Oakes, J. (1986, September). Keeping track, part 1: How schools structure inequality. *Phi Delta Kappan*, pp. 12-17.

(12) Allison, K., Leone, P. E., & Rowse-Spero, E. (1990). Drug and alcohol use among adolescents: social context and competence. In   Leone, P. E. (Ed.), *Understanding Troubled and Troubling Youth* (pp. 178-173). Newberry, CA: Sage Publications.

(13) Meacham, A. (1990). Abuses tarnish adolescent treatment. *U.S. J. Drug Alcohol Depen.*, *14*, 1, 7.

(14) Hamburg, D. A., & Taknaishi, R. (1989). Preparing for life. *Am. Psychol.*, *44*, 825-827.

(15) Slavin, R. E. (1987). Ability grouping and student achievement in elementary schools: A best-evidence synthesis. *Rev. Educ. Research*, *57*, 293-336.

(16) Radziszewska B., & Rogoff B. (1988). Influence of adult and peer collaborators on children's planning skills. *Dev. Psychol.*, *24*, 840-848.

(17) Schuckit, M. A., & Cahhalan, D. (1976). Evaluation of alcoholism treatment. In W. J. Filstead, J. I. Rossi, & M. Keller (Eds.), *Alcohol and Alcohol Problems: New Thinking and New Directions* (pp. 229-266). Cambridge, MA: Ballinger Publishing.

(18) Vaillant, G. E., & Milofsky, E. (1982). Natural history of male alcoholism. *Arch. of Gen. Psychi.*, *39*, 127-133.

(19) Charuvastra, C., Rehmar, R., Paredes, A., "et al.". (1989). Drug-free therapeutic community: a ten-year follow-up. *Addict. Behav.*, *14*, 343-345.

(20) Brizer, D. A., Maslansky, R., & Galanter, M. (1990). Treatment retention of patients, referred by public assistance to alcoholism clinic. *Am. J. Drug Alco. Abuse.*, 16, 259-264.

(21) Business Research Publications. (1989). Facing the future: cost looms as the big issue in treatment. *Subs. Abuse Rep.*, *XX* (ISSN 1040-4164), 1-2.

(22) Schuckit, M. A. , Schwei, M. G. & Gold, E. (1986). Prediction of outcome in in-patient alcoholics. *J Stud. Alco.*, *47*, 151-155.

(23) Emrick, C. (1975). A review of psychologically oriented treatment. *J Stud. Alco.* *36*, 88-103.

(24) Bruning, J.L. & Kintz, B. L. (1977). *Computational Handbook of Statistics.* Glenview, IL: Scott, Foreman and Company.

(25) Stephens, R. (1972). The truthfulness of addict respondents in research projects. *Int. J. Addict.*, *7*, 549-558.

(26) Hesselbrock, M., Babor, T. F., Hesselbrock, V., "et al.". (1983). Never believe an alcoholic? *Int. J. Addict.*, *18*, 593-609.

(27) Pettinati, H. M., Sugarman, A. A., DiDonato, N., "et al." (1982). The natural history of alcoholism over four years after treatment. *J Studies Alcohol*, *43*, 201-215.

(28) Thurstin, A. H., Alfano, A. M., & Nerviano, V. J. (1987). The efficacy of AA attendance for aftercare of in-patient alcoholics: some follow-up data. *Int. J. Addict.*, 22, 1083-1090.

(29) Schwartz, I. (1989). (In) *Justice for Juveniles: Rethinking the Best Interests of the Child.* Lexington, MA: Lexington Books.

Index

4029